PRAISE FOR

A TRANSPLANT FOR KATY

"A disturbing exposé of the dysfunctions in our health care system, told through the story of one young woman's tragically foreshortened life. *A Transplant for Katy* touches on the vexed issue of how treatment decisions are made in America. Rather than being directed precisely by science, Fabregas portrays the liver transplant program at UPMC as motivated by ego, greed, wishful clinical thinking, and good intentions gone very awry."

— **THERESA BROWN**
Staff Nurse and *New York Times* Opinion columnist;
Author of *Critical Care: A New Nurse Faces Death,
Life and Everything in Between.*

"When a beautiful young woman agrees to a daring experimental liver transplant, she doesn't know that the line between medical progress and her surgeon's ambition may be blurry. *A Transplant for Katy* is emotionally rich, intriguing and of historical importance, sounding warning bells for doctors and patients alike."

— **MARSHALL ALLEN**
Reporter for ProPublica, New York

"A compassionate, poignant story of the efforts of the world's foremost transplant surgeon to break through formidable scientific barriers to save the life of a beautiful young woman. Readers of *A Transplant for Katy* will learn about a complex, challenging medical specialty while sharing the heartbreak of a great surgeon and a courageous young woman."

— **CYRIL H. WECHT, MD, JD**
Forensic pathologist and former
Allegheny County Coroner

"I could not stop reading. I am a physician, living kidney donor, and medical researcher (but not in transplantation). I want to say to Katy and the Millers, "My profession failed you. I am sorry."

— **WILLIAM L. FREEMAN, MD, MPH, CIP**
Program Director, Northwest Indian College Center for Health
Human Protections Administrator
Northwest Indian College

"In telling this story of a failed liver transplant, Luis Fabregas, one of the best health journalists working the beat in newspapers today, reveals how ego and money taint modern medicine's commitment to the Hippocratic Oath. *A Transplant for Katy* is an unflinchingly honest, nuanced portrayal of how a bright, promising young woman's life was cut short after she was drawn into an ambitious new liver-transplant protocol. Going deep behind the facade of one of the nation's most revered hospitals, Fabregas shows the venal institutional politics, financial pressures and ethical shortcomings that infiltrated a noble quest to better the science of organ transplants. *A Transplant for Katy* is a nonfiction tale that shows hubris and human folly as starkly and sadly as any Greek myth does, with a novelist's eye for the quirks and foibles of the surgeons who oversaw Katy Miller's unnecessary demise. It should be required reading in any medical school to teach the next generation of surgeons how arrogance and greed can corrupt their profession's promise to put their patients first."

— **JORDAN RAU**
Senior Correspondent, Kaiser Health News

A TRANSPLANT FOR

KATY

Heartache and Betrayal

in the Transplant Capital of the World

LUIS FABREGAS

Fourth River

PRESS

Pittsburgh, Pa.

ISBN-10: 0615672310
ISBN-13: 978-0615672311

Cover design: Melanie Wass
Author's photo: Justin Merriman
Cover photo courtesy of Miller family

To my late grandfather,

Carlos M. Suarez,

who instilled in me a love of writing

"**Facts are the enemy of truth.**"

Miguel de Cervantes

Contents

1

A good feeling

Roger Miller stepped on a half-smoked cigar and hurried down the gravel driveway that circled his home. He jumped into his blue Saturn, squinting at the morning sun. His wife, Kathy, waited in the front seat. Their daughter Katy sat in the back, ears plugged into her iPod, mind on another planet.

Without traffic, it would take Roger 90 minutes to reach the city hospital. Two hours tops, if there were backups on Route 28, a state highway that runs parallel to the Allegheny River. By the time they made it back home, it probably would be nighttime. "Who wants to spend all day on the road," Roger thought, his calloused hands on the steering wheel.

"I have a good feeling about this," Katy shouted to her mother, the way people speak when music is blasting in their ears. Her forehead was pressed against the window, her eyes fixed on the sky.

There were other things Katy Miller would rather be doing on this late summer day. She had to hit the college bookstore to buy her exercise physiology texts for the fall semester. She had to come up with another excuse to brush off Brad, the friend of her brother Jason who'd given her, out of the blue, an expensive tennis bracelet.

This much Katy knew: the last thing she wanted to do was spend another morning – another day – in a doctor's office.

Katy had no choice. Over the last three months, she had been crippled by constant bloating and severe pain in her belly. The bowel movements never seemed to stop. Katy was forced to stay home and skip shopping trips with her mother. She ignored the constant calls from Brad, unwilling to confess she was too sick to go to dinner or a movie. Her pediatrician referred her to a gastroenterologist, who told her she had colitis, a swelling of the large intestine. *Colitis? I can deal with that.*

Meals became a struggle. Katy would press on her stomach to dull the pain. She pushed her plate away, excused herself and curled up on her bed, crying in silence because she wanted no one to know. She'd tried to read, praying the pain would go away.

It was the gastroenterologist who first had a hunch. Let's hope this isn't something more serious, he'd told Katy. He was the one who'd send them to a Pittsburgh hospital for answers. He was the one who put them face-to-face with the liver specialist.

The doctor had turned up an illness Katy never heard of – primary sclerosing cholangitis. The disease attacks the liver's bile ducts, a part of the body no one ever talks about. People talk about the heart, the stomach, even the gallbladder. *What the hell are bile ducts?* They are the tiny tubes that move the dark green fluid that makes digestion possible. The illness makes the bile ducts constantly swollen, so inflamed over time that they harden and form scar tissue. Once Katy's bile ducts became fully clogged, her skin would turn yellow and her strangled liver wouldn't be able to function. *Yellow skin? That sounds gross.* If her liver couldn't work, Katy would only have one choice: a transplant.

Katy Miller was 19, one of eight children raised by a coal miner and a stay-at-home mother who had dreamed of becoming a beautician. As a recent graduate of Marion Center High School, Katy knew little about medicine, much less about organ transplantation. She was a volleyball captain, a gymnast, homecoming queen, a student council member – not someone familiar with the intricacies of the medical world or the vast workings of a health care machine like the University of Pittsburgh Medical Center.

She'd been here just three weeks before. The word "transplant" had been mentioned in passing by one of the doctors she met, Dr. Paulo Fontes, an accomplished Brazilian surgeon. *Liver specialist. Surely he must be good.* Fontes had once been interviewed for the Discovery Health Channel for a segment on organ transplantation titled "Transplant: Kill or Cure?"

He had been more than encouraging. He assured Katy and her family it could be five or 10 years before she needed a new liver. She wasn't sick enough to need one. The transplant may have been on the minds of doctors, but at least it was a faraway option. Years, he said, it will be *years*.

Was he telling the truth? Not three weeks had passed when the phone rang at the Millers' home in Creekside, Pennsylvania, a tiny borough with just over 300 people. Kathy Miller answered the kitchen phone and listened. A woman identified herself as a nurse at UPMC. There was an important question she wanted to ask: *Would Katy and her family please come back to Pittsburgh for a second meeting?* Transplant chief Amadeo Marcos wanted to meet Katy.

Katy's mother wondered what a transplant chief could possibly want.

"Three weeks before they're telling us she doesn't need a transplant and now they want us to come back?" Kathy Miller said years later, her voice weary and monotone.

An American flag flew over the hospital's driveway as Roger Miller pulled into Montefiore hospital. The 13-story building, awkwardly located atop a steep hill, once catered to Jewish patients who were fed kosher food on hospital trays and prayed with visiting rabbis. Jewish doctors in the early 1900s trained at Montefiore, shut out of other hospitals; they embraced a practice of caring for patients regardless of where they came from, who they prayed to, or how much money they had.

Montefiore was now the epicenter of Pittsburgh's world-famous transplant program, named after the man known as the father of transplantation. *The Thomas E. Starzl Transplantation Institute.* That's quite a mouthful, Katy thought. The city of steel mills, with a reputation for black skies and gritty laborers, had been known since the 1980s as the go-to place for transplants: kidneys, livers, hearts. The omnipotent Starzl was the capital's king.

Katy and her parents walked into the hospital lobby and made their way down a long hallway, past a loud lottery machine in the gift shop and a beauty shop advertising $75 perms. They entered the transplant clinic, across the hall from a display of vintage prescription bottles, blood pressure cuffs and black-and-white photographs of the hospital's history.

"Look at those poor people," Katy whispered as she approached a receptionist. She saw people in wheelchairs, others attached to oxygen tanks carried in tote bags. They had yellow skin, yellow eyes. Katy didn't know it at the time, but they were people like her, with rotting livers and uncertain futures.

Yet, for now, Katy felt safe, healthy and alive, comforted by the presence of her parents. Her oldest sister, Shelly, was there, too. They were fourteen years apart, but they were close, almost inseparable.

A woman ushered them into a small conference room, away from the yellow people. Katy examined the white walls, covered with posters of liver diseases and pictures of the human anatomy. She pulled out a Nora Roberts book and tried to read. A few feet away, her parents talked about the ride back home and made plans for dinner. Roger wanted homemade pork chops. Kathy wanted to stop at a restaurant, she didn't care which one.

When Dr. Marcos walked in, Katy was instantly startled by his handsome appearance, more soap opera star than transplant surgeon. Marcos was slim and athletic, with shaggy brown hair. He swam an hour a day at the Pittsburgh Athletic Association, and it showed. When he walked the hospital hallways, sometimes in tailored Italian suits, women stared and made small talk. He responded with a polite nod and a deep stare into their eyes.

"How was the drive?" Marcos asked the Millers, the reality of the meeting not far behind. Their faces were somber and expectant. He wore a white lab coat, green surgical scrubs and a killer cologne that Katy immediately liked.

He pulled up a chair and sat near Katy.

"You are a very good candidate for a new protocol we have here at the transplant institute," he said.

A protocol? Katy didn't quite get it. What was that supposed to mean?

Within minutes, Marcos seduced Katy with words her family would never forget.

"A new liver now can save your life," Marcos said. "Trust me. If you get this transplant, you will live a long life."

Katy fell silent, lost in thought. The words stung, but no one spoke. Marcos' bold pitch – a transplant *now* – was a departure from what Katy heard three weeks ago. Sure, Katy had primary something or other, but she was nowhere near being deathly sick. Dr. Fontes had made it clear the wait for an organ would be long. *It will be years.* Why the change of mind?

The way Fontes had explained it, only the sickest patients rose to the top of the organ waiting list. People were prioritized based on strict rules created by the United Network for Organ Sharing, a nonprofit under contract with the federal government. Liver transplant candidates were assigned a numerical score based on a system that determined their risk of dying within three months. The score, called MELD, ranged anywhere from six to forty. It was based on patient values for bilirubin, a fluid made by the liver; serum creatinine, a chemical waste product; and INR, or the blood's ability to clot.

More than 16,000 people were already on the waiting list and just over 6,000 surgeries would be done that year. Just as soon as they'd get their new livers, more people would be added to the list. Katy could have been added to the list, but her name would be alongside nearly 11,000 other new additions, including almost 1,500 in the geographic region that includes Pennsylvania. Her wait would be long. On average, people in her age range wait more than two years for a new liver.

But who cared, anyway? Katy's liver functions were irregular, but they were not fully deteriorated. *I still have a liver, for crying out loud.* As Fontes explained it, her name would have to be added to the list of people already waiting. That made sense to Katy and her family. She had endured pain, chills and bloating, but she wasn't dying. She could certainly wait two years, and who knows how much longer.

Marcos had a different story. A transplant *now*, when Katy was young and healthy, would come with significantly higher odds of survival. If all worked as planned, she wouldn't be subjected to a lifetime of anti-rejection drugs and their harmful side-effects.

Kathy didn't say much during the meeting; mother's intuition had kicked in. She knew her daughter's life had been jolted by illness, but the thought of a liver transplant, something so drastic, so foreign, made her uneasy. How can you go from colitis to needing a transplant, she asked herself. She felt a strange rush of emotions.

Yet the offer from Marcos was hard to pass up. His words were methodical, seductive and strangely comforting. With a thick but charming Spanish accent, he described the basics of the plan – nearly obliterating Katy's immune system and fooling it into accepting her donor's organ as her own.

It's called tolerance, he said.

The plan's mastermind was none other than Starzl, the 80-year-old pioneer who had performed the first human liver transplant at the University of Colorado on March 1, 1963. *Isn't this the Thomas Starzl Transplantation Institute?* Starzl had been way ahead of most of the field's trailblazers, doing the first liver transplant four years before the South African surgeon Christiaan Barnard would catapult to fame after performing the world's first heart transplant. While Starzl's initial attempt failed, he succeeded four years later, when he performed the world's first successful liver transplant in 1967.

Kathy had many questions. *Starzl, eh? Was he even around, or was he dead? They don't name medical institutes after people who are alive, do they?*

Starzl. The name was strange and foreign-sounding. It was an Austrian name that meant "little man" in Viennese dialect. How ironic. The little man, who had arrived at the University of Pittsburgh in 1981, turned into one of medicine's greatest names. He found a way to redirect the body's blood supply so he could take out a sick liver and replace it with a healthy one. In doing so, he transformed medicine and he transformed Pittsburgh. With Starzl as its chief architect, Pittsburgh became a mecca of organ transplantation, where more than 12,000 transplants were performed in a twenty-year span.

By the time Katy Miller came along with her liver illness in 2005, Starzl had been out of the operating room for more than a decade, yet still was obsessed with this final project. *Tolerance.* Its success would lead to the Holy Grail of transplantation: giving people new organs without subjecting them to heavy doses of harmful anti-rejection drugs. The benefits seemed obvious: a patient could get a new liver and avoid the nasty drugs that in Starzl's early days had threatened to ruin the field of organ transplantation.

Katy could be one of those patients. She could savor adulthood simply by joining Starzl in his quest. She could be part of medical history, and in turn, come away alive with someone else's liver, tricked into thinking it was her own.

The Millers' meeting with Marcos was not meant to be a discourse on Starzl and his achievements. Instead, Marcos spoke to the family about the crippling effects of immunosuppressive drugs, used to stop the body from its natural response to the new organ.

With a standard transplant, Katy would be subjected to high doses of the drug tacrolimus, the gold-standard of immunosuppression in liver transplantation. But tacrolimus, approved in 1994 and known by the brand name Prograf, would not be free of side effects. It can cause a litany of complications: headaches, tremors, diarrhea, high blood pressure, high cholesterol, nausea, stomach pain and abnormal kidney function. Clinical studies described on the drug's website show that up to 22 percent of patients taking Prograf develop insulin-dependent diabetes. At its worst, too much Prograf can lead to infections and lymphoma, a type of cancer.

Headstrong and ambitious, Starzl had spent the last part of his career plotting a plan to get rid of those problems. Sure, he could slice and cut and sew a liver into a patient, but what good would that be if the body, in a furious reaction to the invasion of a strange organ, mounted an aggressive attack against it?

The standard way to treat transplant patients had been to inhibit their immune systems with high doses of immunosuppression. Transplant recipients could then leave the hospital soon after the surgery, without experiencing early rejection of their new organ. That strategy had failed. Starzl had figured out that giving less anti-rejection drugs wasn't necessarily bad. Instead, giving less immunosuppression would activate the body's natural immune response. A battle between donor cells and recipient cells would take place, causing the immune system to go haywire in an attempt to kill the foreign donor's cells. The immune system eventually would get tired of fighting, and accept − or tolerate − the donor cells as if they had been there all along. *Tolerance.*

Starzl had it all figured out. He tried several ways to make tolerance happen and, after failing over the course of several years, he came up with a way to nail the problem. This time, recruiting Marcos to perform the actual surgery, Starzl crafted an intricate plan that he was certain would counter and eliminate the instinctive reactions of the immune system: Before the transplant, the recipient would receive a blast of antibodies, followed by an infusion of white cells from the donor, capped by high doses of Prograf.

The doctors aspired to enroll ten patients in the first round. Katy would be the first. All patients, Marcos told Katy, would receive a liver from a living donor. Katy would have to find a donor − if someone she knew was willing to give up a part of his or her liver. *Do you know anyone who would be willing to do this for you, Katy? A brother, a sister?*

Marcos spoke quickly and convincingly. The liver, he explained, had the dubious distinction of being the most underappreciated organ in the body. Unlike the pancreas, kidneys or any other solid organ, the liver can regenerate on its own from as little as 25 percent of its tissue. Like some lizards that lose their tails, half a liver can grow into its full size within a couple of weeks.

Marcos talked up Katy's age. She was nineteen. At such a young age, Katy faced a lifetime of potentially toxic doses of Prograf. Taking the drugs for such a long time could put her at a higher risk of side effects, Marcos said. *Tremors, headaches, high blood pressure, diarrhea, nausea, constipation. Cancer.*

Katy absorbed every word in silence. The potential for complications scared her. And the chance of not having to endure them seemed like a no-brainer. Why wouldn't she like what she heard? Marcos promised what she wanted: a normal life back in college and the chance to get married and have her own family. She could get a transplant *now*, and forget about her illness once and for all.

Katy smiled and asked Marcos if she had to make a decision right away. *Think about it, Katy. Talk to your mom and dad. And don't forget to think about a potential donor. That's really important, Katy.*

Everything Marcos said seemed to make sense. *A transplant now.* Katy left the room and walked past the yellow people. This time, she didn't look at them. She wouldn't dare think what it would feel like to have skin like that. She couldn't possibly imagine what it would be like to be so yellow. *That looks so gross. Poor people.*

Katy didn't have to think about it for very long. By the time she made it to her father's car, her mind was already made up.

"He seems to be really smart, don't you think, Mom?"

"I don't know what to think," Katy's mother said. "All that talk about a transplant now. It sounds like a lot."

"Oh Mom, he makes a lot of sense," Katy said. "Didn't you hear all that stuff about those nasty drugs? I don't want to put up with that. No way."

"I think a transplant sounds like a pretty big surgery. Do you really want to go through that?"

"I wouldn't see why not," Katy told her mother. "The transplant seems like the way to go."

"What makes you so sure?" her mother said, her brow knitted tightly. "You need to think about this."

"Mom. C'mon. Do you really want me to take all those drugs and get even sicker?" Katy said as she settled in the back seat. "The doctor is right. This is the best option I have right now."

□ ❏ □ ❏ □ ❏ □

I drove my car on the gently sloped, gravel driveway that circled the Millers' home in Creekside – the same place where Katy Miller's journey to the transplant center had begun several months before.

It was early spring, but the sun had been beating on me during the hour-long drive, and I was drenched in sweat. My assignment was to interview a young woman who'd undergone a liver transplant at the University of Pittsburgh Medical Center. I'd been told she was enrolled in a special program to wean patients off immunosuppressive drugs. Her name was Katy Miller, and she was a college student who liked volleyball. I knew little else about her.

I walked up the steps to the house and knocked on the door. Katy's mother, Kathy, greeted me at the door. She was skinny, with droopy eyes and short brown hair. I offered my business card and told her a photographer from the newspaper would be coming along in a few minutes.

I looked around the dining room and noticed a bookcase with photographs of the Millers – a big family of four sons and four daughters – and a stack of books on a corner desk. I had been there two minutes when Katy walked in.

She held a textbook in her hand, and flashing a smile, told me she was studying for a test. She was enrolled in the physical therapy department at Indiana University of Pennsylvania, a 15-minute commute from her house.

I sat at the dining room table and pulled out my notebook. Katy stood at the other end and asked me what it was like to be a reporter. She liked to write, she told me. I told her that to be a good journalist you also have to know to ask the right questions, at the right time. You often have to ask probing questions and be assertive, something she balked at. She didn't like to be mean.

We talked for a while about her interest in sports – volleyball, basketball, cheerleading. Her voice initially was low and sweet, almost as if she were a little girl. I kept looking at her, thinking, "Did this girl really have a liver transplant?" Her skin was radiant, her eyes full of life. Her beauty was almost intimidating.

She sat across from me and loosened up. She turned energetic and spoke with much more strength than someone who had experienced severe liver damage.

Katy described her illness as a temporary nuisance that she had conquered with the transplant four months earlier, on Nov. 1, 2005. "I can move on now," she told me. Her confidence was such that I suspected she'd been coached by the public relations staff at UPMC to say the right thing. That wouldn't have been out of the question; after writing about medical issues for a Pittsburgh newspaper for nearly a decade, I was well aware that liver transplantation was the most treasured specialty at UPMC. The program's image was important to its leaders, and the success of Katy's case surely would be viewed as a colossal achievement.

Katy pulled out a brown duffel bag with brown straps that looked like a backpack. She placed it on the table and unzipped a side pocket. She pulled out two plastic prescription bottles. "This is it," she said. "Want to see?" They were filled with tacrolimus pills, the anti-rejection drug she took to stop her immune system from attacking her new liver.

She showed them to me as if she were showing me candy, as if she wanted me to take one of them and taste it.

Katy asked me for a favor. She wanted to make sure that, when I wrote about her, I would mention her sister Shelly, who donated part of her liver. Shelly was the big sister, the one who put her own life at risk for the sake of her little sister, and Katy believed she deserved recognition in a story about her transplant. I assured her I would mention Shelly.

Nearly two hours later, I walked out of the Miller home, happy with my interview, promising to call when the story was published. The newspaper I wrote for was not sold in Creekside, so I told Katy and her mom that I would mail a few copies. I got in my car and turned on the air conditioning. I took another look at Katy's house, the rows of trees surrounding the property and wondered what it would be like to live so far from the city.

I pulled away and started the long drive to Pittsburgh.

2

Transplant boom

In the mid 1950s, Miami displayed an indisputable glitzy surface. The Rat Pack and Elvis Presley crooned at the city's ritzy hotels along South Beach. Movie stars and politicians jammed the Fontainebleau and the Eden Roc, monuments to excess that sprang up like jewels amid beaches lined with palm trees.

The influx of Cubans was a few years away, and Miami had morphed into the hottest tourist destination for Middle America. The city became a symbol of hope and prosperity. Miami also became a landing place for future doctors who were in demand throughout the nation. With world wars behind them, Americans had turned their attention to better living, medical research and technology. Postwar optimism ruled.

For a young doctor from Iowa named Thomas Starzl, Miami represented not so much a paradise, but a place where he could make a decent wage to support to his young family. Starzl had just finished medical studies in Chicago and Baltimore and was hungry for adventure and eager to sharpen his skills as a surgeon.

He'd make $300 a month at Jackson Memorial Hospital, slightly more than what the average American made at the time. The job provided exactly what he wanted: the surgical experience that can only be had by working in an emergency room busy with crime victims and bullets-riddled bodies.

Settled in the city with his wife and young son, the man who once considered becoming a priest stayed away from the trendy night clubs and devoted his free time to surgical experiments on animals. Starzl yearned to master the art of cutting and sewing a broken body. In med school, he had studied the heart and the brain, the kidneys and the lungs. Something that he couldn't quite explain drew him to the liver – bloody, thick, rich and mysterious.

Starzl found that animals such as dogs provided the best opportunity to probe and explore the liver, its veins and its tributaries. He set up a simple laboratory in an empty garage across the street from Jackson Memorial Hospital. Dog cages lined the garage, filled with the smell of feces and urine.

Starzl and his wife had collected mutts from the city pound and poisoned them with chemicals to make them diabetic – giving them an illness Starzl hoped he could reverse with an experimental surgery. He cut the dogs open and performed a surgery known as the portacaval shunt aimed at diverting blood flow around the liver. It was a procedure he'd learned from another surgeon to reroute the portal vein so that the dark blood it carried wouldn't clog the sick arteries in the liver. The surgery failed. The dogs became emaciated, lost their hair and suffered brain damage. Starzl, either because of innate stubbornness or unsatisfied scientific curiosity, plowed ahead. He continued to slice and dissect dogs in the garage, using instruments and supplies from the nearby hospital. Ever so gingerly, he managed to remove the liver from some of the animals, an operation known as a hepatectomy. Some of the dogs lived for twelve to twenty-four hours after the surgery.

The achievement of taking out the dogs' livers delivered an inevitable conundrum: could they be replaced with a healthy one? No one had ever done such a surgery before. The word "transplantation" had hardly been used in medicine.

"New ideas seldom have the simplicity of a switched on light bulb," Starzl would write in his 1992 memoir, "The Puzzle People."

Starzl left Miami in 1958 and returned to Chicago, where he had attended Northwestern University Medical School. He had spent so much time doing surgeries, he'd developed acute anxiety because he feared he would fail patients if he couldn't save them. He would review the steps of a surgery over and over to make sure he wouldn't make a mistake.

He would make more mistakes, however, in his first attempts to complete transplant surgery in sickened dogs at Northwestern. The dogs died during the operation or a few days after it. Starzl was so frustrated, he pondered a career change and considered abandoning surgery to enter private practice. His mentors were persistent; they recognized Starzl's potential and encouraged him to push ahead and apply for a government grant to study transplantation.

In meetings with the selection committee of the prestigious Markle scholarship, Starzl suspected that his plan to achieve liver transplantation would be spurned. It was an unrealistic goal, he figured, because even if transplantation could be done, there was no way to halt the foreign organ's inevitable rejection by the recipient's angry immune system.

"I asked them to have a lot of patience," Starzl said years later, recalling his meetings with the Markle committee.

Starzl began experiments to cool and preserve livers awaiting to be transplanted. He immersed the anesthetized dog in an ice bath and, when that didn't work, ran a cold saltwater solution into the organ through its portal vein. He conquered another roadblock – maintaining the dog's circulation and avoiding vein blockage – by using plastic bypass tubes to reroute the blood supply during the surgery. Eventually, Starzl and his colleagues reported eighteen dogs with survival greater than four days, with one animal living 20 ½ days.

If transplantation were to become a medical reality, Starzl was poised to be the one to do it. When Starzl was a little boy in LeMars, Iowa, his father was convinced that his son had a higher purpose in life.
R. F. Starzl was correct.

Starzl had a good deal of exposure to hospitals and surgeries from a young age. His mother was a nurse who had worked with an orthopedic surgeon and had great admiration for surgeons. When he was in junior high school, Starzl came in contact with Dr. Wendell Downing, who allowed the boy to watch surgeries and gave him anatomy lessons.

"I was allowed in the operating room at a very young age," Starzl said years later. "I think my destiny was determined early."

Starzl left Chicago for Denver in 1961, where administrators at the

University of Colorado and the Denver VA Hospital were eager to launch an organ transplant program.

Before embracing liver transplantation, Starzl began a series of kidney transplants, a surgery first done in Boston in December 1954. To preserve the donated organs, he used the method he had developed in Chicago, infusing them with a chilled fluid. Five of six patients who were transplanted survived a year, and four survived more than twenty-five years.

On March 27, 1962 at the University of Colorado, Starzl performed the first human kidney transplant at Denver. Less than a year later, on March 1, 1963, he made the first attempt to replace a human liver. The surgeons spent several hours slicing open a three-year-old boy's chest, only to find his liver encased in scar tissue. The boy bled to death.

His death, and that of three other patients, pushed Starzl away from more liver transplants. Instead, he hunted for better anti-rejection therapy, looked for better ways to procure organs, and examined the role of tissue type in transplants.

On July 23, 1967, he performed the first successful liver transplant on a nineteen-month-old girl named Julie Rodriguez. She survived more than a year.

Starzl was on his way to transforming medicine. By taking on the human liver, an organ so complex that no one had dared touch it, Starzl galvanized the medical community worldwide.

He arrived in Pittsburgh in 1980 after a shakeup at the University of Colorado that prompted him to resign. His timing was perfect: Starzl arrived at the same time that University of Pittsburgh leaders were trying to build a multi-hospital academic medical center.

Two administrators there, Dr. Thomas Detre and Jeffrey Romoff, had begun the work with an overhaul of the University of Pittsburgh-affiliated psychiatric hospital, called Western Psychiatric Institute and Clinic. They were wildly successful, turning Western Psych from an anemic hospital with hardly any medical residents to a powerful player with a $60 million budget in the early 1980s – more than six times what it had been in 1973.

Detre and Romoff had bigger plans. They turned their eyes toward other hospitals affiliated with the University of Pittsburgh, including Presbyterian University Hospital.

Romoff, described by some colleagues as arrogant and ruthless, had smarts and business acumen. He knew that to make money and survive, a medical center needed to have the right mix of doctors and medical specialties.

Romoff set his eyes on Starzl, who had been hired by Dr. Henry Bahnson, the chairman of surgery. Bahnson was a star surgeon in his own right and had trained Starzl during a surgical internship at Johns Hopkins University in Baltimore. Bahnson had been best man at Starzl's first wedding in 1954.

Starzl's first four liver transplants in Pittsburgh failed. He retreated and focused his interest on cyclosporine, a drug whose anti-rejection effects had been discovered in Switzerland and Starzl had studied in Colorado.

Cyclosporine caused kidney damage, but Starzl discovered it could be used in combination with steroids to prevent rejection in kidney transplant patients. Starzl's drug cocktail eventually worked; it enabled surgeons to decrease the dosage of cyclosporine to minimize its nasty side effects.

The discovery led to what historians and medical journals describe as the "Golden Age" of organ transplantation. Sick patients clogged Presbyterian Hospital and more than 100 kidney transplants were done in one year. Starzl was on his way to becoming a medical icon.

Detre and Romoff capitalized on Starzl's talent and fame and, perhaps more important, his ability to attract patients to Pittsburgh from all over the world. Pittsburgh, known to the rest of the nation as a smoky city and the land where Super Bowl and World Series champions were made, became the transplant capital of the world. It was an unofficial title that came with the promise of much-needed revenue for the fledgling medical center.

Several members of the Saudi royal family and some Middle Eastern leaders trekked to Presbyterian hospital to get liver transplants. At UPMC's height in 1990, Starzl and fellow Pittsburgh surgeons performed 471 liver transplants, more than any other center in the country. Starzl became as popular as some of Pittsburgh's most acclaimed personalities, including Fred Rogers, beloved host of the children's television show "Mister Roger's Neighborhood," and Art Rooney, founding owner of the Pittsburgh Steelers.

Starzl described the era as a gold rush with a shortage of gold miners. Medical students, mesmerized by organ transplantation, found their way to Pittsburgh, hungry to learn from Starzl and build their own transplant programs. At one point in the early 1980s, Starzl had trained nearly ninety percent of all transplant surgeons in the United States.

By 1991, though, Starzl had enough. He retired from clinical practice, a decision that meant Detre and Romoff needed a capable successor to continue the path to growth and profitability. The natural choice was Dr. John Fung, who had been with the system for years, and as Starzl's protégé, seemed poised to carry out his legacy.

If Starzl was the king of transplantation, Fung was the heir apparent. He was thirty years younger than Starzl, but Fung managed to make a name for himself. Fung was a prodigy who graduated from college at nineteen and went to the University of Chicago, where he obtained both a medical degree and Ph.D. One of Fung's most significant achievements, in June 1992, was the world's first baboon-to-human liver transplant. The recipient was a thirty-five-year-old man dying from hepatitis B. The baboon was chosen partly because it was capable of resisting hepatitis infection. The man, whose identity was kept secret, lived seventy days with the baboon's liver inside him. Starzl and Fung attributed the man's death to the proportions of a mixture of four anti-rejection drugs. The operation – and a second one in January 1993 – had failed, but the fact they were performed at all brought worldwide attention to Pittsburgh.

Fung teamed up with Starzl and others to refine the use of the anti-rejection drug tacrolimus, then called FK-506. The doctors led clinical studies that showed the drug was far less toxic to the kidneys than cyclosporine. The drug's development, and its subsequent approval by the Food and Drug Administration in 1994, cemented Pittsburgh's reputation as the go-to place for an organ transplant.

Fung became the voice of UPMC in 1996 when he spoke passionately at federal hearings about the nation's organ allocation system. He argued for changes in a federal policy that distributed donated organs to patients based on where they live, instead of their level of sickness. Fung's campaign stimulated new organ allocation rules.

"It made people realize that transplantation wasn't a boutique thing to do, that it was basically trying to help patients who would have otherwise died," Fung said years later.

Fung had emerged from the shadow of his mentor, but his career would soon take a detour. Starzl and Fung weren't the only ones on a path to change organ transplantation. Another man would soon make his grand entrance.

□ □ □ □ □ □ □

The television news report jolted Ken Schuler. The Virginia man never watched the local news but, one winter evening in 1999, he sat in his living room and put on WHSV TV-3. A reporter was interviewing the father of a thirty-nine-year-old woman who was dying from a rare liver disease. Without a new liver, Deborah Parker could die within six weeks. Someone help my daughter, the father pleaded on camera.

Schuler had a hunch he could help. He turned to his wife, Bettie, and proposed that he could donate part of his liver.

"Had she been drowning in a river, I would've stopped to rescue her, not much difference giving her my liver if she's dying," said Schuler, 47, an artist who made a living telling stories in pencil drawings of the wildlife and woods he could see from the windows of his home.

Schuler had never met the woman from Virginia Beach, but within minutes, he was flipping through the phone book for the TV station's phone number. He wanted to talk to Parker's father. His blood was B-positive, same type as Parker. He was eager to help.

Over the next several weeks, Schuler underwent dozens of medical screenings and tests. He met with more psychiatrists than he did other doctors, and he eventually received clearance for the historic fifteen-hour surgery. He had full confidence the surgery would be successful.

Some people thought Schuler was crazy; no one in the world had ever donated part of his liver to a total stranger. Reporters called from CNN and from as far away as Japan.

The surgery saved Parker, a mother of three children. She lived another eight years before she died from kidney failure.

"She got to see her daughter get married," Schuler told me years later. "I would do it again in a heartbeat."

The surgeon who scrubbed in to do Schuler's surgery on April 19, 1999, was a 36-year-old man named Amadeo Marcos. Schuler had a hard time understanding the doctor's broken English. Marcos was born in Cangas del Narcea, on the north coast of Spain, and at the age of five moved with his parents to Caracas, Venezuela.

Amadeo Marcos was an enigma to his patients, his subordinates, even to his closest colleagues. No one really knew why he got into medicine, though some speculated that it was as a way to spite his rich father, with whom he had a rocky relationship.

Marcos seemed perfectly suited for a field that demanded heart, not just smarts. From his early days at Hospital Vargas in Caracas, Marcos formed strong bonds with his patients. Linton Guadalupe, a man in his twenties battling gastric cancer, was one of them. Marcos went to Linton's hospital room several times a day and often changed his patient's dressings, even if they didn't need to be changed. Sitting in a wheelchair, Linton would sneak outside the hospital to smoke cigarettes with Marcos, a notorious smoker.

When Linton eventually left the hospital, he never forgot Marcos and often came back to visit. Marcos enjoyed his company.

But Linton's cancer came back, and he died a few months later. Marcos was angry, devastated and confused, and refused to return to work. One evening he left the hospital, determined never to come back.

Fellow residents went to Marcos' home, eager to help him. They pleaded with him to return to the hospital. A mentor offered a key piece of advice: There is a fine line between caring *for* patients and caring *about* them, he told Marcos. Never cross that line, the mentor urged. The mentor spoke with force: Take care of patients and don't get attached to them. The words made sense and, from that moment on, Marcos turned his attention to the complexities of surgery – and to organ transplantation. He chose a career in the United States, away from the political instability of Venezuela, a country then mired in economic crisis and rampant with corruption.

Marcos arrived in the United States in 1995 during a remarkable period in the country's medical history. The AIDS pandemic had reached a full decade. Stem cells from human embryos were being isolated for potential use against diseases. Mammograms were becoming widespread to screen for breast cancer cells.

There also was a boom in organ transplantation. Sick people clogged the handful of transplant centers in the country looking to replace their sick kidneys and livers. From 1988 to 1993, the number of liver transplants doubled to more than 3,400. To address the demand – and the short supply of organs – doctors began using live adult donors for pediatric surgeries.

Marcos landed a fellowship at the Medical College of Virginia in 1996. He brought solid references from top doctors such as Dr. Roger Jenkins, chief of transplantation at Beth Israel Deaconess Medical Center, the teaching hospital affiliated with Harvard Medical School. Marcos had worked at Beth Israel for two months, hired after the departure of a prominent group of surgeons.

Dr. Robert Fisher, himself a pioneer in organ transplantation, supervised Marcos in Virginia. Fisher immediately liked Marcos. He found the young surgeon bright, articulate and always sharply dressed.

Unlike Pittsburgh, where surgeons had access to organs from as far as West Virginia, Fisher and his team did not have access to many organs, limited by the organ allocation process and the scarcity of donors. People on the waiting list were dying faster, unable to get the organs they desperately needed to survive. Doctors turned to live donor surgeries as a way to give patients a shot at life. The surgery's potential prompted Fisher to send Marcos to Hannover, Germany, so he could learn about it from Dr.

Christoph Broelsch.

Broelsch had been working in the United States when he became the first surgeon to transplant part of a dead donor's liver into a child. He also had split a cadaver liver in two and transplanted the halves into separate children. But it was the surgery that Broelsch performed in 1989 at the University of Chicago Medical Center which garnered the most attention – the nation's first live-donor liver transplant.

The world watched the surgery in awe, captivated by the young recipient – a 21-month-old girl named Alyssa Smith from the San Antonio suburb of Schertz, Texas. Alyssa had biliary atresia, an often fatal disease that was blocking the tiny bile ducts connecting her liver to the intestines. Doctors put her on a transplant wait list, but told her parents that since she was on a normal growth curve she would likely have a long wait. Alyssa could die waiting.

Doctors in San Antonio told Alyssa's mother, Teri Smith, about the experimental, live-donor transplant. The option came loaded with ethical questions because it placed a perfectly healthy person – the donor – under the knife. Teri, who was in her twenties, didn't care. She had learned as much as she could about the surgery and didn't think twice about saving her daughter.

On November 29, 1989, Broelsch and his team spent 13 ½ hours in the operating room completing the dual surgeries. They removed Alyssa's sick liver and replaced it with about a third of her mother's liver – her left lobe. Journalists from around the world covered the story. First Lady Barbara Bush called to offer her well-wishes.

"Once you've given someone a big piece of your heart, it's easy to throw in a little bit of liver," Teri Smith told reporters.

Alyssa's surgery wasn't perfect. Surgeons inadvertently tore her spleen and had to remove it, putting her at higher risk for infections. She later underwent a second surgery to stop bleeding and recovered. Alyssa graduated from college in May 2010 with a degree in social work and took a job in Raleigh, North Carolina.

"She was just a mom saving her little girl," Alyssa told me years later.

Marcos was a quick study. He worked long hours at the Virginia hospital, sometimes finishing a liver transplant only to jump into another surgery, perhaps a kidney transplant in an adjacent operating room. Patients like Schuler, who wound up donating his liver to a stranger, had full confidence in Marcos. They admired his skill and his bedside manner.

Schuler saw Marcos many times after his surgery. He grew fond of the surgeon and was especially happy that, with his help, Deborah Parker had been nursed back to health.

Marcos charmed his patients. He played jokes on them, and to retaliate, they pulled pranks on the doctor. Transplant recipient Bruce Wenger tricked Marcos into thinking that a small wire in his hand was a small tube that was supposed to be attached to his skin to drain bile. "Look, doctor, it just fell out," Wenger said. Marcos turned white before Wenger exploded in laughter.

Wenger was one of Marcos' first patients in Virginia and the first in the United States to get a liver from a non-blood relative, his wife. The surgery prompted reporters from around the world to call Marcos for interviews. His star was rising quicker than he'd ever expected.

On a live chat on CNN in 1999, four months after Parker's transplant, callers praised Marcos for saving the lives of family and friends, and cheered when Marcos spoke about a favorite tradition: calling his patients on the anniversary of their transplant to sing an out-of-sync version of "Happy Birthday."

"I have to admit that I'm a very lousy singer," Marcos said.

Marcos' success and his growing power quickly transformed his way of thinking. While he never stopped caring for his patients, some colleagues said Marcos became arrogant and vain. The mentors who had believed in him were suddenly confused.

"He gave the impression that he was like the Virgin Mary, but in male form," Fisher told me.

Fisher admitted he may have contributed to Marcos' increased feelings of superiority. When they collaborated on research and papers for publication, Fisher allowed some of his underlings, including Marcos, to take lead authorship. It gave them a chance to learn and to become known among their counterparts elsewhere in the country.

Marcos was suave and debonair and that made him extremely popular with women. That got him into trouble. Barely eight months after Parker's surgery, a post-doctoral fellow in the psychiatry department filed a complaint with the Equal Employment Opportunity Commission in Richmond. It was serious charge, alleging that Marcos sexually harassed and assaulted her. It was the culmination of a pattern of abusive and sexually inappropriate behavior over the previous four years.

On the verge of being fired, Marcos resigned from the Medical College of Virginia on March 27, 2000.

"I felt, what a horrible travesty, what a loss," Fisher said later. "He had the capacity to be an incredible individual. But he had many failures."

Marcos' next stop was Rochester, a city in New York not exactly known as a medical hub, but as the home of companies like Kodak and contact lens maker Bausch & Lomb. Rochester may not have been Harvard, but Marcos quickly became an influential surgeon at Strong Memorial Hospital.

His often abrasive personality came through the first time he met Bill Morris, the man in charge of the hospital-based organ procurement organization at Strong. It was about 2 a.m., and Marcos was getting ready to scrub in outside the operating room when someone tipped him off that the donated liver had not yet made it to Rochester. A furious Marcos called Morris at home.

"Where the fuck is that liver?" Marcos screamed. "What the fuck is wrong with you?"

"Where are you?" Morris replied. When Marcos told him he was in the OR, Morris got dressed and drove two miles to the hospital where he confronted Marcos – the first time he had laid eyes on him.

"Don't ever talk to me like that," Morris warned him.

Marcos shot back: "What are you going to do, sue me?"

Marcos wound up reporting Morris to the chairman of surgery, Dr. James V. Sitzmann.

"If he didn't like something, he reacted with hostility, yelling and screaming," Morris said years later. "He was an expert at intimidating people."

Yet Marcos, married to anesthesiologist Cristina Roosen, showed evidence of being a family man and a doting father. His son was crazy about wrestling and Marcos treated him to a match of the World Wrestling Federation held at the War Memorial in Rochester. Marcos brought a camera so the boy could take pictures. He fed him french fries and wiped the boy's ketchup-covered mouth with his own napkin, according to Morris, who wound up becoming a close friend of the surgeon's despite the early friction. Marcos retained his ties to his homeland of Venezuela; he traveled to Caracas often to visit family and even to go to the dentist.

As was the case in the rest of the nation, patients at Strong found themselves in the midst of a nationwide shortage of organs. The overachieving Marcos grew restless. He began doing what some surgeons considered a measure of last resort: using organs that might be considered unsuitable by other surgeons because of the donor's age or health. Doctors refer to them as "extended-criteria organs," even though some transplant pioneers can't agree on what constitutes an optimal donor organ. This much they know: an organ's eligibility for transplantation can be affected by the donor's age, the cause of death or if there was exposure to an infectious disease. The ideal donors up until then had been people younger than forty years old.

Surgeons at Strong quietly began to use extended-criteria organs in 2000. No one knew about it until four years later, when the New York Department of Health disclosed an investigation of the hospital. Health officials would not say if Marcos had been involved, but found ten violations in Strong's liver transplant program. In one case, a patient required two additional transplants after receiving a liver from a donor with incompatible blood type. In a second case, surgeons failed to justify the reason for using an extended-criteria organ on a patient who had a favorable, short-term survival rate without the transplant and wound up with post-surgical complications. Even more, the hospital failed to complete a thorough pre-operative work-up on a patient to determine the need for transplantation. In other cases, patients weren't told they were getting organs from questionable donors.

The health department's findings spread like wildfire. It didn't take much for Marcos to realize that his job was in jeopardy. He needed to get out – fast. All signs pointed to Pittsburgh.

□ □ □ □ □ □ □

In the small fraternity of organ transplant surgeons, all dots connect to one person: Thomas Starzl.

Starzl led a period of unrivaled activity in organ transplantation, and his name became synonymous with the field. To know Starzl was to know medical royalty.

Amadeo Marcos didn't know Thomas Starzl. But he knew John Fung, and that was just as good.

Fung completed his surgical training at Rochester and had turned down repeated offers to chair Strong's transplant department. Marcos, on the other hand, had once before attempted to make his way into Pittsburgh by applying, unsuccessfully, for a highly coveted transplant fellowship.

In the summer of 2002, Marcos called on Pittsburgh again. He'd been making frantic calls to colleagues at transplant centers across the country asking about potential jobs. Marcos was at risk of losing his job at Strong Memorial Hospital and eager to find a new one.

Fung knew of Marcos. They were not friends, but they had smoked cigarettes together at transplant meetings. Marcos boasted that Fung was a close colleague. Fung was gracious enough to listen. Within weeks, Marcos met with key leaders in Pittsburgh, including the chairman of surgery, Dr. Tim Billiar; the hospital's top administrator, John Innocenti, and Starzl, who was retired from the operating room, but typically was consulted on important research and administrative matters.

The last word on his hiring, however, would come from Jeffrey Romoff. He was now president and CEO of the medical center and had built a network that included the city's best-known hospitals, including Children's Hospital of Pittsburgh. Romoff liked Marcos and offered him $500,000 a year and additional incentive payments, according to a story in The Wall Street Journal. He would report to Fung with the title of clinical director of transplantation. Marcos accepted it over an offer from the Texas Liver Center in Houston that reportedly promised a much higher salary.

Marcos became the transplant program's new rock star. He made no secret of his goal to boost the number of live-donor liver transplants, an emerging specialty that was sure to address a stagnant number of donated organs. The number of live-donor liver transplants shot up within a year of Marcos' arrival, to twenty-five in 2003 from four the year before.

As Marcos' star rose, Fung's faded. Fung publicly denounced Pittsburgh's focus on profit, not research. He'd been ordered to boost transplant volume and with good reason: hospitals bill insurers up to

$200,000 for every transplant-related admission.

"The only metric that the people in this program seem to see is how much they are billing," Fung told me at the time. "It's an approach that is somehow tunnel vision. People are so focused on doing more cases that no one is writing about it so others can learn about it. It doesn't recognize that people have talent that goes beyond making money."

By 2004, the number of liver transplants using deceased donors in Pittsburgh was plummeting, to less than half what it had been in the late 1980s. Transplant fellows were unable to meet training requirements to complete forty surgeries because too few livers were coming to Pittsburgh.

A watchful Romoff took notice and wasted no time pushing Fung aside. He jetted Fung six time zones away to Sicily, where the university had established a transplant hospital aimed at making available its medical expertise to anyone in the world, regardless of where they lived. The $58 million facility, called Istituto Mediterraneo per i Trapianti e Terapie ad Alta Specializzazione, resembled a five-star hotel and gave UPMC the potential of boosting its profits by as much as $20 million a year. In addition to transplants, Pittsburgh doctors in Italy began doing heart bypass surgery and cancer surgery.

Fung, an ocean away from the mothership in Pittsburgh, was cut off from making decisions on the transplant program's day-to-day operations. Transplant fellows were instructed not to call him if they experienced complications or had questions about a case.

"It's clear the University (of Pittsburgh) wouldn't be involved in (transplantation) if it wasn't financially solvent," Fung said years later.

Marcos was different. He was in awe of Starzl and took very

seriously his opportunity to expand the program. Marcos gave Romoff what he wanted – a big-time commitment to resurrect Pittsburgh as the once-dominant transplant mecca. Marcos seemed hungry for power, with a drive and ambition that rivaled Starzl. It was exactly what Romoff wanted: someone pushy and aggressive to light a fire under the transplant program.

Marcos moved with confidence through the halls of Presbyterian hospital. While initially he was reserved, he began to throw occasional temper-tantrums, especially when a liver expected to come to Pittsburgh from another city ended up going to another transplant center. To nurses and aides, his knowledge translated into arrogance. The minute he stepped on the transplant unit, everyone knew he was there. He was loud and often short with many of those he encountered.

"Do you think we should order an ultrasound?" a nurse asked upon seeing a patient's chart.

"That's for me to decide," he replied.

It was as if Marcos were playing the part of a hard-boiled, die-hard Starzl. Like Starzl, Marcos smoked cigarettes, a habit he gave up during his first months on the job. He walked the hallways often dressed in expensive Armani suits, constantly chewing Nicorette gum. Nurses spoke in hushed tones about his love of expensive cars. His everyday car was a Porsche Cayenne, but if he felt like it, he came to work in a red Ferrari.

While Marcos was never as grandiloquent as Starzl, he spoke with a loud voice and did not so much give orders as demand them in an instant. Nurses looked away or feigned busyness when he walked in, afraid they couldn't produce what he wanted. If he asked for something, they'd better make it happen.

In 2003, the Pittsburgh transplant program – and by extension, Marcos – drew the ire of surgeons across the country who had uncovered that Pittsburgh surgeons knowingly used extended-criteria organs that were unsuitable for transplantation. A committee of the United Network for Organ Sharing found that using those organs, which had a high probability of failing, put Pittsburgh at an unfair advantage for receiving organs to replace them. The practice bumped patients up the waiting list and the UNOS committee noted the Pittsburgh program had logged an unusually high incidence of patients re-listed for transplantation. Surgeons in the same organ distribution region as Pittsburgh were furious; they were not getting organs for their patients and accused Pittsburgh of abusing the organ allocation system.

"If you want to use marginal organs, you have to know how to use them, when to use them and who to use them for," Dr. Cosme Manzarbeitia, a transplant surgeon then working at Albert Einstein Medical Center in Philadelphia, told me in April 2004. "You can't be ridiculously aggressive. You can buy a used Mercedes or you can buy a 1925 Ford abandoned in a parking lot. They're both used cars, but one is going to run and the other one is not. There's organs and there's organs."

The use of extended-criteria livers, it turned out, had led Pittsburgh surgeons in 2002 to put 7.2 percent of their patients, or twelve people, back on the waiting list within a week of their transplant. Indeed, the patients wound up at the top of the list over other patients. Surgeons complained that Pittsburgh was siphoning organs for those patients. Even more, those patients often improved, but instead of giving back the organs to other centers, Pittsburgh was keeping them for other patients.

UNOS responded by creating a payback rule in the regional area that included Pennsylvania, West Virginia, Delaware, New Jersey, Maryland and Washington, D.C. Under the rule, Pittsburgh owed a liver to another hospital each time it got one to replace a failed organ.

Pittsburgh administrators denied they'd done anything wrong. They said some extremely sick patients were re-listed for a second transplant as an added precaution, but were removed from the list when they improved.

Starzl at the time did not address the payback rule, but spoke about efforts by some surgeons to avoid a practice he called organ wasting.

"Every time you throw out an organ that can be transplanted, it's very apt to cost a life," Starzl said. "So there's been a national movement socially driven to try to make better use of the organ supply because there's an enormous death rate from people who die while waiting."

Marcos remained mum about the issue. It was summer 2004 and Fung, still the transplant chief, was growing exceedingly dissatisfied with the program. In July 2004, he made the surprise announcement that he was taking a job as chief of surgery at The Cleveland Clinic. Although shocking to those who viewed Fung as a Starzl loyalist, his departure cemented Marcos' new role as transplant chief. If there was a national search to replace Fung, no one knew about it. Marcos was in. He had Starzl's blessing and nothing else mattered.

Marcos' promotion was big news in a transplant town. I wrote a front-page story that Marcos found offensive. The story quoted patients who praised Marcos but also provided details about the sexual accusations in Virginia and the use of extended-criteria organs in Rochester. Marcos was not one to read newspapers, but someone gave him a copy of the story, and it was clear he didn't like it. Over a two-year period, he ignored my repeated requests to speak with him about the future of Pittsburgh's transplant program.

That changed in the spring of 2006. I'd become acquainted with Starzl who, as the son of a newspaper editor, always took a liking to journalists. I met Starzl in his office to interview him for a story about his eightieth birthday and purposely mentioned my one-way feud with Marcos. In a Starzlism of sorts, he intervened and fixed the problem, feigning no involvement.

A few weeks later, I received a call from the public relations officer at the University of Pittsburgh asking if I was interested in writing a story about a liver transplant protocol. Marcos had agreed to talk to me about it.

Better yet, a college student from outside Indiana, Pennsylvania, was the first patient in the protocol, and she was willing to be interviewed and photographed. I didn't understand the implications of the protocol.

Until I met Marcos for the first time.

□ ❑ □ ❑ □ ❑ □

Amadeo Marcos walked in wearing blue scrubs and black Gucci loafers and shook my hand firmly. I greeted him in

Spanish, my native language, too, as we sat in a conference room at UPMC Montefiore. A public relations officer positioned herself within earshot, pulled out a notebook and took notes as if she were the one writing the story.

Marcos joked about doing the interview in Spanish. I laughed politely, but we both agreed English was more practical for business.

"Spanish is better for poems," Marcos said.

Over the next hour or so, Marcos gave me a medical lecture, schooling me about liver transplants, organ shortages and the hardships of immunosuppressive drugs.

"Even though we don't have enough organs, and I don't know that we'll ever do, it's what we do and how the patients do once they get the transplant that's having the biggest impact," he said. "If you were to have any transplant, from kidney to lung to heart, after five to ten years you're going to have significant consequences, not of the transplant that can be working well – but of the medicines you are on for immunosuppression."

The anti-rejection drugs, despite preventing rejection of the transplanted organ, were the surgery's number one enemy. Starzl in his early career had faced and described such roadblocks. As he wrestled with the technicalities of the surgery, Starzl identified what he considered a serious barrier to organ transplantation. He referred to them as "new diseases in the transplant recipients' population." Steroids, given to patients to suppress the immune system, were the culprit. "The steroids caused redistribution of fat and other changes that were so cosmetically deforming that they could be interpreted as nature's revenge for defeating its purpose of rejection," Starzl wrote in his memoir.

Starzl described the undesirable and harmful side effects of the steroids – the organ recipient's face ballooned and a buffalo hump appeared between and just above the shoulder blades. He wrote of children no longer growing as they were supposed to; patients experienced cataracts, stretch marks, weakened bones and nasty infections of the lungs and brain. Something had to be done.

Marcos spoke about immunosuppression and its destructive side effects with the same disdain Starzl had displayed years before. The drugs were so nasty, they wreaked havoc with a person's glucose, blood pressure, bone density. Many liver transplant recipients were forced to undergo yet another transplant to replace the weakened kidneys.

"So what is tolerance?" Marcos asked, speaking in run-on sentences. "In simple terms, it is to have the body accept the transplanted organ in a way as if its own. You kind of mimic a transplant between identical twins. You will not require immunosuppression."

Tolerance. That had been Starzl's mantra, Starzl's driving force over the last forty-five years. Starzl's fascination with tolerance went all the way back to his days at the University of Colorado, where his career took off in the early 1960s as an associate professor of surgery. It was then that forty-six transplant patients received kidneys from relatives.

Seven of those patients, who received little immunosuppression four weeks before their transplants, lived up to forty years taking no immunosuppression after the surgery. Two others received minimal doses of immunosuppression. Yet some patients died, an observation that confused Starzl and others in his team.

"That was a very unusual experience," Starzl had said. "We

couldn't understand what we had accomplished."

In 1992, Starzl and his team of researchers dug deeper into the Colorado kidney transplants. They examined the thirty patients with the longest survival by performing biopsies of their lymph nodes, skin and other tissues. They found that the patients, despite having had surgeries three decades earlier, had traces of original donor cells. Donor lymphatic cells – T-Cells and B-cells – were supposed to have died a few months after the transplant, but they were still alive. Why were they still present thirty years later?

It was a light-bulb moment in the quest to ensure a patient could survive following organ transplantation. There was no sense in mastering transplant surgery if the new organ wound up being annihilated by the patient's immune system. Starzl was convinced there was a way of creating the right balance between donor cells and recipient cells so they could live in peace. He called the concept "microchimerism."

Chimerism – a term derived from the fire-eating monster Chimera in Greek mythology, with the head of a lion, the body of a goat, and the tail of a serpent – captivated Starzl.

"This was so attractive to him, this concept of having people off immunosuppression," Marcos told me.

Marcos spoke with candor, and it was clear he had assumed the role of leader of Pittsburgh's transplant program – a role that once belonged solely and squarely to Starzl. Marcos displayed assertiveness and confidence, looking me straight in the eyes and often repeating the same words over and over.

"Let me know if it gets too complicated," he told me when he talked about B-cells and T-cells, the two main type of lymphatic cells in the immune system.

Once Starzl had discovered microchimerism, the obvious next step was to replicate the process, even if some of the Colorado patients had not been weaned off the anti-rejection drugs. Nine of them had been drug-free and that was good enough for Starzl.

The first thought seemed like a natural solution. To achieve tolerance, Starzl proposed taking bone marrow cells from the donor and infusing them into the transplant recipient in the hours after the surgery. Bone marrow transplantation, in which healthy new cells are given to a patient, had worked in patients with illnesses such as leukemia or lymphoma. Those new cells – stem cells that can develop into any type of cell in the body – find a way to be accepted in the recipient's body. This plan, however, involved giving patients a lot of immunosuppressive drugs on top of the bone marrow cells. It provided patients some benefit but not quite what surgeons had expected.

"We were giving a lot of immunosuppression, the same immuno-suppression that almost every center in the nation uses today. Three drugs at the same time at high doses. So we were not letting the immune system of the recipient interact with those cells that were coming," Marcos told me.

Starzl concluded there was no need to kill the entire immune system for donor cells to co-exist with the recipient's cells. There was no need to be Draconian. There was a purpose for the interaction of donor cells and recipient cells and it was best if nature took its course. Starzl had used three terms to explain the process: activation, exhaustion and deletion. The cells come together and react to each other. The recipient cells become exhausted by the battle. They then disappear – deleted – or die.

Starzl's rationale wasn't just a fleeting idea. He vowed to put his discovery into action. He laid out his strategy in two papers he co-authored with Dr. Rolf Zinkernagel, a Swiss immunologist and 1996 Nobel laureate.

The papers, published in 1998 in *The New England Journal of Medicine* and in 2001 in *Nature Reviews: Immunology*, explained that tolerance could occur by allowing the natural immunological reactions to take place. Better yet, tolerance could be achieved by encouraging rejection, something that was completely counter to common wisdom about organ transplantation.

In the latter paper, "Transplantation tolerance from a historical perspective," Starzl and Zinkernagel explained how to achieve tolerance clinically – by controlling the amount and timing of the anti-rejection drugs, known as tolerogenic immunosuppression. They concluded tolerance could not happen if patients were given high doses of anti-rejection right after the transplant because the immune system would be too weakened to mount its attack. Fewer anti-rejection drugs were better.

Starzl recognized the approach hinged mostly on finding the right time to activate the recipient's immune system – much like refueling a race car. If you refuel after the race, you won't win. You have to refuel at the right time and learn to manage the fight that ensues, careful not to destroy the liver, or to crash the race car. If you timed immunosuppression right, you can win the race – and eventually reduce immunosuppression.

Over the next several years, putting this approach into action became Starzl's obsession. The first attempts did not succeed: recipients were getting too much immunosuppression, a misstep that interfered with the crucial battle between the immune system and the army of foreign donor cells.

From 2001 to 2004, doctors in Pittsburgh performed more than 1,000 transplant surgeries, most of them kidneys, using a standard of care that was the precursor to the guidelines used on Katy. It involved giving patients shots of antibodies right before the transplant to kill white blood cells that would launch an attack against the new organ, followed by small doses of immunosuppression after the surgery. Donor bone marrow cells also were given at the time of transplant, or shortly after, an effort equivalent to blowing cold air on a fire – it doesn't put out the fire in the recipient's immune system but cools the house so it doesn't burn down.

The surgeries succeeded, but the doctors struggled to wean patients off the anti-rejection drugs on a consistent basis. Starzl was certain the protocol's timing could be adjusted – and enhanced. He worked day and night to come up with a strategy. In 2004 he met with Zinkernagel in Innsbruck, Austria, and crafted a plan that altered the timing and manner in which the donor cells were given to the recipient.

The plan, as Marcos described it to me step by step, was "the ultimate clinical protocol to achieve constant and maximum immunosuppression reduction." It was quite an endorsement, and he was intent on selling it to me.

Instead of giving donor cells to the recipient after the transplant, the infusion of donor stem cells would take place twenty-one days before the surgery. The time element was crucial because it allowed three weeks for the interaction between donor and recipient cells to take place. The recipient also would be pre-treated with the drug campath, which destroys T-Cells and B-cells but not precious stem cells, and low doses of tacrolimus. By the time the actual transplant took place – with yet another infusion of the donor bone marrow cells present in the new organ – the reaction had occurred and tolerance would be achieved.

"This will change transplantation," Marcos said. "This will change our outcomes and the long-term survival and function of grafts of our patients. I think it will change transplantation. That is Dr. Starzl's main interest."

"How do you know it will work?" I asked.

"It *has* worked," he responded. "It has worked to some extent. We just haven't been able to control this process as we can now."

The protocol was no fluke. It had been forty-five years in the making – but Marcos wanted to make sure I got the message right.

"This is forty-five years of his work," Marcos said about Starzl. "To think that he invented transplantation and made this a reality…"

Starzl and Marcos concluded that using the protocol in liver transplants with live donors would be more effective because in deceased organ donation, doctors only have twelve hours to identify a recipient and time for pre-treatment is minimal. Using the protocol on patients who had a live donor would be done within a more predictable environment and would give doctors an extra three weeks to manipulate the recipient's immune system.

"The goal of this is not to totally stop immunosuppression. The goal of this protocol is to reduce it as much as possible, still preserving good organ function," he said.

Still, some patients would go from taking three pills a day to taking a pill once a day.

"That's like taking nothing in reality," Marcos said. "You have no idea how many pills these patients take."

Starzl, convinced that he had nailed the protocol and that it had the best chance at good outcomes, conceded it wasn't necessary to try it on kidney patients, as had been the practice with earlier tests of tolerogenic immunosuppression.

Marcos, it turned out, was the one who persuaded Starzl to move forward. Marcos was eager to start right away. Using live donors typically involved using healthier recipients, and surgeons could control exactly when the surgery would take place.

Marcos could taste victory. There were plenty of people in need of a new liver. Including Katy.

□ ❑ □ ❑ □ ❑ □

On Sunday, April 2, 2006, Marcos sent me an email, composed entirely in Spanish, regarding a story I wrote for the *Pittsburgh Tribune-Review* about Starzl's new tolerance protocol:

Dear Luis,
I am very impressed with your article published today. In reality,

you are the first to report on this therapeutic modality that is going to change the future of the world of transplantation. Your article is extremely true and complete. I am impressed that you were able to capture all the tolerance concepts that on occasion are difficult to pass on even to members of the medical community. Upon reading your article, I feel the same way as I did in 1998 when I performed the first live-donor liver transplants in America. On that occasion it was the press that was in charge of disclosing that new advance in the field of transplantation. Today it is you who is doing it. Please receive a warm embrace from a Latin counterpart who hopes to have many future and productive interactions with you.

Amadeo

3

A promising life

Katy Miller was blue when she came out of her mother's birth canal at Indiana Hospital on March 31, 1986. Her umbilical cord was wrapped around her neck and a doctor had to force oxygen down her windpipe. Her parents always joked that was the reason why Katy was the smartest of their eight children.

Katy's mother, Kathy, was only fourteen when she met her future husband at a fairground in Indiana, Pennsylvania. Eighteen-year-old Roger Miller, cocky and handsome with a head full of wavy hair, slapped her on the behind. Kathy gave him a dirty look and ignored him.

Kathy's cousin, Judy, had other plans. She'd set her eyes on one of Roger's friends, Ray, who didn't have a car. Roger had a pickup truck, and his buddy begged him to let him use it for a date with Judy. Roger agreed, but only if he would drive and Judy would bring Kathy. Ray had no other choice. The four teenagers went to a drive-in movie, and ever since that summer night, Kathy has never had eyes for another man. It wasn't that she'd been eager to fall in love. In fact, that was the furthest thing from her mind. But she found Roger to be bold and independent, the type of man she didn't want to lose.

The couple married on September 27, 1965. The small ceremony was held at the home of a minister, an acquaintance of Roger's family. Roger, fresh out of Army boot camp, wore a military uniform; Kathy wore a blue suit. They didn't have money or time for a fancy reception. Roger was on a fifteen-day leave and within days left the young bride for a year-long deployment in Germany. Kathy, young and penniless, moved in with her parents. She took a job as a cashier, determined to save money. By the time Roger came back, they had enough cash to buy twenty-three acres from Roger's brother in Creekside.

There are no big highways in Creekside, only winding roads surrounded by trees. It's the type of town where properties are tucked into patches of woods and the nearest gas station is five miles away. The tiny borough butts against Indiana, the hometown of screen legend Jimmy Stewart. When strangers ask where Creekside is, residents always mention Indiana. Even a sign on Creekside's border along Route 422 welcomes drivers to Indiana, the Christmas tree capital of the world.

The newlyweds' money stretched only so far, and they had enough to build the bottom part of their house – a two-room basement that several years later Katy and her youngest sister turned into a bedroom. It was as if the sisters had their own apartment, with the convenience of having mom's food every day. Upon the birth of their first child, the couple finished off the brick home with three bedrooms.

Roger and Kathy didn't plan on having more than a few children.

It just happened that way. When Roger ended his stint in the military, he tried to get back into the coal mining industry, but jobs were scarce, and he settled for a seasonal factory job. Kathy stayed home in those early years, tending to three little ones – Bucky, Shelly and Bryan. Roger, eager to work on his own, partnered with his brother-in-law to form an auger mining company. Nearly a decade later, Kathy got pregnant again. And again. And again. Five more little ones: Kristy, twins Josh and Jason, Katy and Ashley. By that time, Roger was successfully managing three augering companies.

"I never became a millionaire, but I raised eight kids on it," Roger said later.

Roger and Kathy toyed with several name for Katy. Their final choice didn't match the baby when they saw her for the first time. "Why don't you just use your name and take out the letter H?" Roger suggested to his wife. Kathy immediately agreed, even giving Katy her middle name, Diane. So Katy Diane it was.

Shelly, the oldest, became her mother's unofficial assistant. Shelly cleaned, changed diapers and cooked, even though she was a tomboy who loved to play in the woods and splash in the creek with her brothers. Even when her little sisters came along, Shelly never played with the dolls her mother stored in a basement toy box.

The Miller home buzzed in the mornings. Roger woke up at four and left no later than five. He felt the pressure of having eight little mouths to feed and many times wouldn't get home until late evening. Kathy set up a hairstyling shop in the basement and word spread in the neighborhood that she was giving decent haircuts for a few bucks. Neighbors and relatives showed up, sometimes without notice. Shelly helped her mother, giving shampoos and unrolling perm rods. Shelly, who was fourteen when Katy was born, took a special liking to the little baby with the olive-colored skin and curly black hair.

Little Katy loved movies and *"The Little Mermaid"* captured her budding imagination. Curious and adventurous, the little mermaid lived in an underwater kingdom and longed to be part of the human world. Katy watched the movie constantly and begged her mother to name her little sister after the mermaid Ariel. Her mother didn't want to hear it and named the baby Ashley. Even without the name Katy lobbied for, Ashley and Katy became close.

There was plenty of bickering among the Miller kids. They fought over basketballs, board games, and the last cookies in the Tupperware container. While the twins ganged up against Kristy, lifting her by the neck, feet dangling in the air, they never touched Katy. It was as if Katy had managed to shield herself from the mischievous hands of her brothers. When it was time to do chores and their mother ordered them to clean their bedrooms, do dishes, or take out the garbage, Katy stayed away from the commotion. She was slick and quiet and burrowed in a corner with a book. She soon became known as the golden child. Katy could do no wrong. She was everyone's best friend.

Down deep inside, a competitive spirit burned inside Katy. She was quiet, but eager to take on her brother and sisters. Just after school one fall, the Miller kids got off the bus at the bottom of the hill that led up to their house.

"I'm starving," Katy told Jason as they walked to the house.

"Me too," her brother said. "I am so hungry, I could eat a hundred chicken patties."

"No way, Jason," she said. "I bet I can eat more than you."

Thus began Creekside's first-ever chicken patty-eating challenge. Katy and Jason ran up the steps to the house, threw their book bags on the floor and headed straight to the kitchen. Katy opened the freezer and reached for a box of frozen chicken patties. Jason found a loaf of bread. Kristy egged them on, partly amused and partly unsure if her brother and sister would pull off the challenge.

Jason turned on the oven and reached for a cookie sheet that he placed on the kitchen table. Katy yanked the chicken patties out of the box and lined them on the tray.

They shoved the tray in the oven and waited. By the time the patties were done, the kids had assembled a line of hamburger buns on the table. The kitchen suddenly had turned into a war zone. Plastic bags, chicken patty crumbs and spilled lemonade covered the floor. Katy quickly placed each patty on a bun, closed it and pressed it down.

"Everyone ready?" Kristy chimed. "At the count of three. One. Two. Three. Go!"

The battle began. Katy sat at the table and ate each sandwich with speed and purpose. She wasn't just eager to beat her brother, she was hungry. With machine-like ability, she downed one patty. Then two. Three. Four. Jason trailed behind. If he slowed down, Katy would get bloated much faster than him. Yet, for the next thirty minutes, Katy maintained a comfortable one chicken patty lead over her brother. By the time it was over, Katy had downed seven patties. Jason ate six.

"I got it handed to me," Jason said later.

Their mother wasn't amused by the gorge-fest. She walked into the kitchen and looked around in disbelief, trying to make sense of the leftover buns and the half-eaten patties on the table.

"What the hell are you guys doing with all those damn chicken patties?" she asked.

Kathy Miller learned patience the hard way. She wanted her kids to succeed and to be kind, studious and respectful, but she also encouraged them to have fun. She pushed her daughters to join a popular cheerleading squad. The girls had dabbled in gymnastics and Kathy wanted them to remain active. They joined the Evergreen Eagles, whose athletes traveled to national cheerleading competitions. The group had just started a pee-wee squad, and Katy joined as a pom-pom girl. She was dedicated and enthusiastic. Coaches set up her first solo routine to the song "Footloose" because Kathy didn't want her dancing to anything too provocative. Katy memorized every move in her routine. She'd been told not to touch her skirt, even though its pleats were being stubborn. They folded up and exposed her behind. In dress rehearsals, Katy straightened the skirt, but the coaches scolded her.

"You're going to lose points if you do that," a coach said.

"I don't want my butt hanging," Katy pleaded. It didn't matter, the coaches told her. No sooner had she started her tumbling steps, Katy's skirt became stuck, but she didn't dare touch it. She completed the entire routine with her behind in full view to spectators even though it was covered with tights. Judges commended Katy for her perseverance. Her family couldn't stop laughing.

Katy qualified for an all-star national competition in Myrtle Beach, South Carolina. She was in seventh grade, and it would be the first time she traveled away from home and the first time the family would see the ocean. The younger kids in the family – Kristy, Katy, Josh, Jason and Ashley – piled up in the family's oversized van, black with teal stripes, which in an amusing coincidence were the same colors as the cheerleading uniforms. Kristy hated everything about the eleven-hour drive. Katy loved every minute of it.

In Myrtle Beach, cheerleading ruled, but Katy discovered an intense connection with the ocean. The water mesmerized her and made her feel free and alive. From that trip forward, Katy vowed that she would one day live by the ocean and marry a handsome man.

The man of her dreams would have to obtain her father's approval. Roger Miller wasn't a hovering father, but he was fiercely protective of his daughters. He was once a young bachelor and knew that guys could be aggressive on the dating scene. That's why, when Shelly started dating, Roger made it clear that he wouldn't tolerate anyone who disrespected his daughter. The first person to discover how serious Roger was about this was Scott McGinnis. Scott went to school with Shelly and wanted to take her out. When Scott showed up at the house to pick up Shelly on their first date, Roger Miller pulled out a handgun. He flashed it in front of McGinnis's eyes and delivered a stern warning on how to treat young women such as his daughter.

The incident did not scare off Scott, who married Shelly with her father's consent. Shelly and Katy remained close, even though Shelly moved 30 miles away. When Shelly and Scott's daughters, Kayla and

Myah, were born, Katy was the first in the family to hold them. Katy regularly spent the night at their house and joined them on beach vacations.

Like her siblings, Katy never strayed far from her family. If she wasn't home, she was likely in school, at a student council meeting or in volleyball practice. During her junior year at Marion Center High, she became captain of the volleyball team. She was loyal to her parents and just about the only time she disobeyed her mother was on the week leading to homecoming night. Katy had been voted homecoming queen and she and her mother picked a gown that she'd wear for the dance. Just four days beforehand, Katy called her mother from the mall. She'd found another dress.

"What about this dress we just bought?" Kathy asked, annoyed, calculating the money she'd spent on the dress.

"I don't want to wear it, Mom," Katy said, and described the new gown, black with shades of fuchsia. "Trust me, you'll like this one."

Katy and her sisters inherited their father's large eyes – brown, sparkling and playful. Katy's were framed by a mane of dark hair that reached her shoulders. Unlike her outspoken sister Kristy, Katy was more reserved. Yet she was deeply intuitive and always spoke with self-confidence.

Katy regularly donated blood. The American Red Cross held drives at Marion Center High, and Katy willingly rolled up her sleeves. At seventeen, she had the wisdom to appreciate the impact of small gestures. Giving blood was a tiny expression of charity that took a few minutes and perhaps could save a life, Katy believed.

Four days after a spring blood drive, Katy received a letter from the American Red Cross. Her mother shuffled through the stack of mail piled up on the kitchen counter and picked it up. *American Red Cross?* Oh, probably a thank-you, she thought. Who knows, maybe they're having another blood drive, and they want Katy to go. She was about to toss the letter in the garbage when something told her to open it. She ripped open the envelope and read. Something about Katy's recent blood donation at Marion High. Kathy read the letter for a second time.

The Red Cross had not been able to use Katy's blood, the letter said. The blood had been flagged after the standard screening tests. Katy's blood was showing an elevated amount of liver enzymes. *Thank you for your blood donation to the American Red Cross.*

Early the next morning, Kathy called a physician in the pediatric practice she'd used for all her kids, Dr. Christina Lubold. The doctor allayed Kathy's fears and suggested a new round of blood tests. When they came back normal, Kathy felt relieved and forgot about the incident.

One afternoon Katy came home from school complaining of a stabbing pain in her abdomen. She had diarrhea and told her mother that her stomach felt as if someone were stabbing her with a pitchfork.

"Mom, I'm scared," she said.

Over the next several days, Kathy treated her daughter's symptoms with Kaopectate, Pepto-Bismol and anything she could think of. Katy was exhausted and her mother was increasingly anxious. This was not fair, Kathy thought. As a caregiver, she was running out of options. As a mother, she was starting to think something else had to be wrong.

"I'm just so tired," Katy said.

The pain persisted. In yet another appointment with Lubold, the pediatrician sensed Katy needed help from a specialist. She referred Katy to Dr. Shirish Amin, a gastroenterologist. Amin was a gentle doctor who immediately liked Katy. He peppered her with questions as he reviewed the records he'd received from the pediatrician's office.

Amin decided to perform a colonoscopy to inspect Katy's colon. The test would provide a detailed look at the entire length of her colon. Amin wanted to find any ulcers, polyps, tumors or areas of inflammation or bleeding. He wanted to provide Katy an answer about her constant pain. In preparation for the test, he ordered his patient to drink nothing but chicken broth and water. The test won't take much more than an hour, he said.

Amin studied the images of Katy's colon flashing on the monitor before him. He'd seen images like that hundreds of times and was all too familiar with the bumpy layers of the colon wall and the prominent, red blood vessels of an inflamed intestine. His diagnosis: colitis, a pesky inflammation that causes tiny sores to build in the lining of the colon. The intensity of the inflammation makes the colon empty frequently, leading to diarrhea, cramps and abdominal pain.

Amin couldn't say what was causing the inflammation, but most doctors rarely have an immediate answer for this type of condition. Most experts blame colitis on an overreaction of the immune system to normal bacteria in the digestive tract. Some studies have shown there could be a genetic predisposition to the disease or environmental factors that contribute to its development. In most people, the symptoms come and go. Others, however, have symptoms all the time. They may have a fever, lack appetite or lose weight.

Amin prescribed prednisone, steroids that he hoped would reduce the inflammation. He ordered Katy to stay away from dairy products. There would be no milk, cheese, butter or yogurt. Katy had never been much of a milk-drinker anyway, so it wasn't something she would miss. Mother and daughter rearranged the timing of their shopping trips. Instead of going to lunch before hitting the stores, Kathy and Katy ate after shopping, in case Katy had to go to the bathroom.

Katy's follow-up blood work troubled Amin. Her liver panel – the enzymes and proteins that give a snapshot of how well the liver is working – had not stabilized. It could be something other than colitis, Amin suspected. He wanted reassurance that he wasn't missing a larger problem.

"We need to rule out anything more serious," Kathy remembered hearing.

To do this, Katy would have to be examined elsewhere. Amin sent her to the best place he could think of: UPMC.

No one in the Miller family had ever needed medical treatment at a large, advanced hospital. Roger and Kathy's eight children had grown up healthy, and their interactions with the medical world were limited to routine visits to the pediatrician.

"They had colds and the flu, but nothing chronic," Kathy said. "They were never in the hospital."

The two-hour drive to Pittsburgh from Creekside was rare, limited to the occasional day trip to Kennywood, an amusement park along the Monongahela River where the Miller kids stuffed themselves with potato patch fries smothered in gravy and rode roller coasters until they were dizzy and exhausted.

The Millers took in the crowded and busy neighborhood surrounding the hospital. There were dozens of college students from the University of Pittsburgh in every corner, some of them in shorts and flip-flops despite the chilly autumn weather. It was hard to find parking, and even harder to find their way around the maze of hallways in the hospital.

Dr. Paulo Fontes, a good-looking surgeon in his early forties, greeted Katy and her mother with a warm smile. He had dark hair and a strong but soothing voice. Fontes was one of about six high-profile doctors in UPMC's liver transplant team.

Fontes had pored over records similar to Katy's since completing a clinical fellowship in Pittsburgh under Starzl in the early 1990s. Katy's recent history – the chronic fatigue, the loss of appetite, the ulcers in her colon and the abnormal liver enzymes – immediately raised his suspicions. All Fontes had to do was order a specialized X-ray to figure out if her bile ducts were narrowed, as he suspected. To obtain the X-ray, called a cholangiogram, doctors insert an endoscope through the mouth, into the stomach and then into the small intestine. They guide a thin tube into the bile ducts and inject dye to highlight them. It was exactly what Fontes suspected.

"It's called primary sclerosing cholangitis," he informed them in one of several appointments.

To Katy and her mother, the name sounded like another variation of colitis. It was not. The illness had a hard-to-pronounce name, and both Kathy and Katy were mildly relieved when they were given its shortened name, PSC, as if that would make it any better.

Fontes delivered an easy-to-understand crash course on PSC. The walls of the bile ducts become so inflamed they develop scar tissue, and the naturally soft walls turn hard. Like a sink clogged with sludge and debris, the bile ducts block and start to shut down.

The blockage builds up bile, the liquid that breaks down fat in food, and damages liver cells. If too much bile collects in the ducts, it starts to seep into the bloodstream. The bile ducts become infected, causing fever, chills and tenderness in the upper abdomen.

The relentless assault of this nasty disease against liver cells ultimately destroys the liver. People with severe liver damage need a transplant, the only known cure for PSC, but typically not until 10 years after being diagnosed. The illness also can lead to bile duct cancer.

"To go from colitis to something so drastic like this? It was hard to understand," Kathy said later.

Fontes dismissed the idea of a transplant. He explained that Katy would have to be sicker and stand in line behind the thousands already waiting. The long wait often prompted patients to find a living donor, often a relative or friend, he said.

Katy left the meeting feeling uneasy about the road ahead. *I have to deal with this now and it will be over.* The more she thought about it and considered her options, the better she felt. *It will be over. I will get rid of this miserable illness.*

For now, doctors at UPMC had a plan to fix her, Katy reasoned. She drove back home, away from Pittsburgh's noisy streets. She felt safe in Creekside. She felt safe in the house her parents built. Most of her brothers, with families and children of their own, had moved to homes within a hundred yards of her parents. It wasn't rare to find some of them at her parents' house at any time of the day or night.

Kathy pulled up the driveway and looked at her house. Her mind turned to the letter Katy had received from the American Red Cross. *Thank you for your donation.* The damned blood donation had started everything. Kathy now found herself conflicted about how to make the best choice for her daughter. The prospect of a transplant rattled her, even if it was years down the road. They are the best doctors in the world, she thought to herself. *She's in the best hands.*

Katy didn't say much when she walked in the house. She went straight to her bedroom and called Shelly.

"We're back from Pittsburgh," she told her sister. "I'm fine."

"Oh, good. What did they say?" Shelly asked.

"They talked about a transplant but they said it could be years away," Katy said. "Hopefully it won't get that bad."

The meeting with Amadeo Marcos would soon change her life.

4

Donors at risk

7 2,288. 72,289. 72,290. The numbers change in real time. They appear in vibrant colors on the website of United Network for Organ Sharing, the federally-backed nonprofit that tracks transplants in the United States. 72,292. 72,293. 72,294. They represent the people whose lives have been shattered by illness and wait for a live-saving organ.

72,299. 72,300. 72,301. On any given day, thousands of Americans wait for kidneys, livers, intestines, hearts, and other organs. They get phone calls in the middle of the night. *There's an organ for you.* They rush to the hospital, only to discover they're incompatible with the donor.

Again, they wait. Sometimes they get lucky. Others die. More than 2,500 people in the United States die waiting for a liver every year. They die waiting because they are either too sick to withstand the massive assault on the body that is transplant surgery – or because they are not sick enough to move up the wait list.

Some people wait days. Some wait months. Others wait years. Katy did not want to wait. Not one year, not five, and certainly not ten. She faced a type of liver disease she believed she could conquer, either with a conventional liver transplant – using a deceased donor – or one in which surgeons used a live donor. Katy wanted a transplant *now* because she wanted to move on with her life.

When doctors at UPMC told her that she would likely have to wait years for a deceased donor, she found the concept of live-donor transplantation intriguing and, in many ways, hopeful. She felt like a breast cancer patient who's told by her doctor that her abnormal tissue can be taken out without destroying her breast. The surgery would save her life and she would move on. Without waiting. She could have the surgery on her own terms. *Now*. Katy did not want to be a number on the UNOS website.

"I want to move on with my life," she told her mother two days after doctors first mentioned the surgery.

Moving on would have its consequences. It would force Katy to consider questions that had saddled the field. The surgery that Amadeo Marcos had just proposed came loaded with ethical and moral quandaries: Was her life worth enough to put a healthy donor at risk of dying? If the donor died and Katy lived, how could she face the rest of her life?

For a would-be donor, the answer always comes easy. Yes, I want to help. Yes, I want to give a piece of me so someone else can live. Katy came from a big family of four brothers and four sisters, which made her list of potential donors much longer than that of the typical transplant candidate.

When they heard Katy was considering a live donor, all of her brothers and sisters stepped up. Immediately. And how could they not? They had to do it for their little sister, the golden child, the one who always managed to stay out of trouble.

Their good intentions quickly faded into reality. The older guys were married and had family responsibilities that made it impossible to spend months away from their jobs to recover from the surgery. Kristy, the most outspoken of the girls, joked that some of her brothers were too big and fat to withstand a surgery like a transplant.

"Their livers are probably huge," she joked.

That left Shelly, the oldest of the four girls, as the most likely candidate. Shelly and her husband, Scott, had two daughters, Myah and Kayla. Katy was almost like a third.

"As soon as she told me what was happening, I knew I would be the one," said Shelly, who looks like Katy, only taller and with shorter, shoulder-length hair. "I would do anything for her."

Shelly and Katy were fourteen years apart but they had the same body structure and weights. Shelly was healthy and didn't have any of the diseases that could rule her out as a donor: high blood pressure, diabetes, cancer or kidney trouble.

"I knew my liver would be the better match," Shelly said.

To get clearance to become a donor and go through a potentially disabling surgery, candidates undergo an evaluation that varies, depending on the hospital they choose. Its purpose is to not just uncover medical problems that could prevent the donor from giving the organ, but also to make sure the donor can endure the operation.

In most transplant centers, the evaluation includes a history and physical examination to look over the donor's vital signs and prior medical history. Potential donors meet with a liver specialist who is not a surgeon but acts as the donor's physician. In some cases, they meet with anesthesiologists who will be in charge of pain management and monitor blood pressure, heartbeat and breathing during the surgery. They also meet with psychiatrists who assess their mental stability. *I'm not crazy, I really want to do this.*

Before signing a consent form, Shelly and Scott contemplated dozens of questions. There were the obvious ones: Who will take care of the girls while Shelly was in the hospital? Who will cook? Who will take them to school? Then there were the questions no one dared think about: what happens to Myah and Kayla if Shelly dies in the operating room?

"I was scared," Shelly admitted.

She met with a transplant coordinator who reviewed a long list of potential problems. Shelly had a fifteen to thirty percent chance of developing a complication, either minor or major. Two out of seven donors were at risk. Most of the complications were likely to be minor but they couldn't rule out something that would require another surgery or some type of extra medical intervention. The most common complication was a bile leak, which resolved on its own without any type of intervention.

"They did a very good job at explaining everything that could happen," she would say later.

The amount of information donors receive prior to their surgery is up for debate. Two extreme and fairly prominent cases, in 1999 and 2002, first focused public attention on the need for a better system to inform patients.

Danny Boone died twenty-one days after donating part of his liver to his brother in North Carolina in 1999. Mike Hurewitz died three days after donating more than half his liver to his brother in New York in 2002. Hurewitz, a fifty-seven-year-old journalist, died after picking up an infection. Boone, who was forty-one, had an undetected liver disease and also died from an infection.

The cases punched a hole in the optimism that had enveloped the live-donor liver transplant field. The number of surgeries nationwide, which accounted for about ten percent of all adult liver transplants, dropped from about 400 a year to about 250.

Dr. Francis Delmonico, director of renal transplantation at Massachusetts General Hospital, spoke about the dangers of the surgeries to transplant surgeons and other physicians at a 2003 meeting of the American Transplant Congress and expressed growing unease over the practice of using live donors.

A living donor is "not just a client or a commodity," Delmonico told the group, according to an article published in the Journal of the American Medical Association.

The backlash against the surgery mobilized reformers and eventually forced UNOS to mandate transplant centers to establish a written living donor consent process.

Donna Luebke, a transplant patient advocate, kidney donor and former board member of UNOS, maintains that the policy is not enough. There are no standards for centers to create an evaluation or consent mechanism. Each transplant center therefore sets its own screening or suitability criteria. Advocates have suggested a federal registry of donor morbidity and mortality. It hasn't materialized.

"No doubt some programs have stepped up to develop living donor policies, educational tools, etc., but nothing really has changed. Nothing nationally. It's buyer beware, donor beware," said Luebke, a nurse practitioner in Cleveland.

In May 2010, a man who donated part of his liver to a sick relative died during the surgery at Lahey Clinic near Boston. The program's director, Dr. Elizabeth Pomfret, had addressed the issue of donor deaths at the same transplant meeting where Delmonico had spoken seven years before.

Pomfret told the gathering that the procedure "is not as easy a thing for a donor to go through," as initially thought. State officials who investigated the donor death did not uncover any problems with the program's quality.

Three months later, tragedy struck again at The University of Colorado Hospital. Ryan Arnold, a thirty-four-year-old-father of three, died four days after donating part of his liver to his brother, Chad.

Chad suffered from PSC, the same illness afflicting Katy. He survived the surgery, turning to a blog to share the agony of losing the brother who was trying to save him.

"I missed you today, Ryan," Chad wrote on one of his entries. "It hurt so much I felt like my heart had blisters on it. God, why do we need death to reawaken what we should already know?"

The Colorado hospital temporarily stopped the live donor

transplant program, same as they did at Lahey, where surgeons have performed the most live-donor liver transplants in the country. An autopsy showed Ryan died from cardiac arrest and suffered from a slightly enlarged heart. Hospital administrators vowed to implement better monitoring of donors after surgery, setting up a machine that sounds an alarm if oxygen levels drop and the patient stops breathing. Even so, Luebke remains unconvinced.

"I will hold firm to my belief that the living are not the solution to the organ shortage," Luebke said.

Some transplant centers appeared to agree. Some of the nation's centers stopped doing the surgeries. Cedars-Sinai Medical Center in Los Angeles stopped doing live-donor liver transplants in 2005 in part because of fear of complications and new organ allocation rules that allowed for better use of organs from deceased donors.

"If one of my patients had a complication…I would feel very badly about it, even if it was only a statistically small likelihood of it happening to someone else," Dr. Andrew Klein, director of Cedars-Sinai's Comprehensive Transplant Center, said in a newspaper story.

Shelly and Scott considered the possibility that something could go wrong. Scott had experienced the death of a loved one in 1996 when his 25-year-old brother, Donnie, died unexpectedly of bacterial meningitis. Scott didn't want his wife to experience the same type of loss.

"I don't want you to lose her like I lost Donnie," Scott told his wife. "You never forget the pain."

Shelly weighed the possibility of losing Katy against the information she was given by her transplant coordinators and doctors. She shuddered at the thought of the medical risks she faced: scars, hernias, pain and fatigue, organ failure and the chance of a transplant – and death. She was forced to ponder how she'd feel if Katy would reject her organ and die. But with every question and every answer, she arrived at the same conclusion. She could not afford to lose her sister.

It was the same rationale that convinced Shelagh Ruane to give part of her liver to her sister Teresa in 2005. Shelagh grew up in Uniontown, about fifty-five miles south of Pittsburgh, but had moved to Charlotte, North Carolina. When she'd come home to visit, she noticed that Teresa was frequently sleeping. After years of drinking, she was showing signs of alcoholic liver disease. The illness causes the liver to get swollen and inflamed, slowly destroying it. The scarring on Teresa's liver prevented blood from flowing through the organ. Instead, blood flowed through the veins of her esophagus, causing its veins to balloon outward.

Doctors warned Teresa that her liver was so diseased, she would likely need a liver transplant. The harshest warning had to do with the long wait. *You can wait for years. You can die waiting.* Teresa's parents, both in their 80s, drove her to the clinic every week, an hour long drive each way, for appointments and checkups.

The strain on her parents became too much for Shelagh to bear from so far away. She told Teresa she would donate part of her liver. The way she saw, it wasn't really her liver. It was God's liver. At night time, she sat in the backyard of her parent's home and prayed.

"Am I doing the right thing?" she asked herself. "Am I interfering with God's work?"

The sisters spent the night before the surgery in a hotel a few blocks away from the hospital. They slept in different rooms, in case they had to use the bathroom at the same time. They went out for a dinner of Chinese food. Just before their meals arrived, Teresa gave Shelagh a bracelet as a remembrance of the bond they were about to share. Shelagh was happy that she had chosen to help her sister. They left the restaurant and hopped in Shelagh's car. As she backed out, the car hit a pole that she hadn't noticed.

"Shelagh! Pay attention!" Teresa said.

Shelagh had been distracted, thinking about the surgery, life and her future. She realized at that moment that, in the great scheme of things, it didn't matter that she had just dented her car.

Both the transplant and Shelagh's donor surgery were a success. But it wasn't long before Teresa started drinking again. Shelagh felt she'd been betrayed.

"That blew our relationship out of the water," Shelagh said firmly. "If you give a present, people are going to do what they want with the present."

Teresa got sick again. Her parents were furious. She died four years after the transplant, alone and rejected by her parents.

Shelagh experienced a bad fate of her own, with several medical setbacks. Pneumonia. An abscess in one of the lungs. Staph infections.

She eventually lost her job and went on disability, prompting a period of self-examination.

"Terri's death was so sad," she said, trying to find a way to explain it. "She died alone. We didn't even tell my mother until Mother's Day the next year."

For every story like Shelagh's, there are stories like the one of Ali Lingerfelt-Tait, a nurse and mother of three in North Carolina. Like Katy, Ali was one of ten. Ten patients had been carefully chosen to enroll in the Starzl-Marcos protocol and Ali also would be one of them.

At around the same time that Katy became sick, Ali began to experience the symptoms of PSC. Ali retained so much fluid, she looked like she was, in her own words, "ten months pregnant."

Ali chose to get listed at two transplant centers – near her home in Chapel Hill, and in Pittsburgh, where she had been assured she would have access to the most experienced doctors in the world. Ali's husband was a primary care doctor, which along with her own background as a nurse, allowed her to ask the right questions. The dual listing offered no guarantees. Ali's blood was O positive, the most common type of the four major blood groups. That meant that she would be competing against the majority of patients on the wait list.

Ali learned as much as she could about transplant surgery and realized it was a complex procedure that came with a multitude of risks. She could reject the liver, she could pick up an infection or she could die on the operating room table. That sort of thing happens all the time, she told herself.

"We're not talking about a tonsillectomy here," she said.

Despite the low odds of getting a liver from a deceased donor, Ali had ruled out considering a live donor, a requirement to enroll in the protocol. Only one person had emerged as a potential candidate – her son, Simon, who was twenty-three. She felt sick at the possibility that anything could happen to him.

"I didn't want to put his life at risk," Ali said about her son. "I knew the dangers of having a live donor. Anything could happen to him. You take a perfectly healthy person and you put them at risk. God knows what could happen. They might nick something or get an infection."

As Ali's wait for a deceased donor extended, she got sicker. Swollen veins in her esophagus and stomach threatened to rupture and cause a large amount of blood loss. She agonized over what to do: Should she go for the live-donor surgery and put her son at risk, or allow her illness to continue its attack, putting her at risk for cholangiocarcinoma, a cancer of the bile ducts? Up to fifteen percent of people with primary sclerosing cholangitis can get that type of cancer.

"Once you're handed that set of cards, it's terrifying," she said.

At a meeting of the PSC Foundation in April 2006, Ali met Katy for the first time. Katy spoke about her successful liver transplant. *Look at me, I feel great.* The encounter gave Ali pause and something more to think about, but she wasn't quite convinced. Days later, a conversation with a relative who was a school psychologist finally convinced her.

"Think about what you'll do to Simon if you die and he has to live the rest of his life wondering if he could've saved you," Ali was told.

Ali said: "I'm his mother and I'm going to sacrifice his life?"

Ali, however, needed to focus on surviving. She postponed a decision, but finally had the transplant on October 17, 2006. As one of the ten patients in the Starzl-Marcos protocol, she didn't go into the surgery expecting to gain full tolerance, and she hasn't. She remains healthy, happy and philosophical about her experience. When I spoke to her, I was impressed by her openness and her willingness to share the lessons she learned. I survived for a reason, she told me.

I asked Ali about Katy. You get a transplant, it's a risk, she said. *This is not like you go on and get cosmetic surgery.* We talked about Katy's enthusiasm, about grief, about life. She spoke about the importance of organ donation, something she continues to believe in. In the end, there were no clear answers about Katy, other than sometimes when you stand on the precipice of death, you take anything you're offered to avoid the fall.

Shelly recognized she didn't have to agree to become Katy's donor. Members of the transplant program told her that she had some degree of control over her involvement in her sister's surgery. She could reject the donor surgery and not put herself through the exhausting physical evaluation, the painful biopsies and the haze-inducing painkillers. She learned donors often back out of a transplant without telling the truth to the intended recipient. They often chalk it up to an unsuccessful match – the wrong tissue type or the wrong organ size.

She didn't have the heart to say no, even though there were several times before the surgery when she could have easily walked away.

"Are you sure you can do this?" Katy asked Shelly when the two were alone at their parents' home.

"Why wouldn't I?" Shelly said. "You would do the same for me, right?"

"Well...I don't know," Katy cracked. "I would really have to think about it."

5

A sexy organ

The liver is the human body's sexiest internal organ, a transplant surgeon once told me. A healthy liver has smooth curves and a soft texture. It is pink and firm with no fat, sharp on one side and well-rounded on the other.

A sick liver is dark, hard and angry. It looks like a bag of marbles, with bumps created by a net of scars that lock together into a lattice. The bumps make the liver seem shrunken and distorted.

Replacing that hardened, clogged filter with a healthy organ is one of the most complicated and demanding undertakings in medicine. Some surgeons call it the granddaddy of surgeries. It is a drawn-out, highly synchronized marathon that takes close to eight hours to complete. From its very start, the liver transplant is a strenuous fight in which doctors peel off the bad liver from the vena cava, the biggest vein in the body. Because the entire blood supply goes through the vena cava before going into the heart, a liver transplant can be a bloodbath.

In patients with cirrhotic livers, the planes between the cava and the liver are slightly inflamed, making it even tougher to separate. To make matters worse, patients with liver disease are unable to clot blood. That makes for a bloodier battle zone and puts surgeons one move closer to death.

To contain and minimize the blood, doctors slice open the body with an electric device they call the Bovie that cauterizes tissue as it cuts the skin. It fills the operating room with the smell of burnt flesh.

Katy's liver transplant would not only be long, it also would be heavily monitored by surgeons at UPMC. The plan called for Katy to get about two-thirds of her sister's liver in simultaneous surgeries in side-by-side operating rooms.

Dr. Amadeo Marcos scheduled Katy's transplant for 7 a.m. on November 1, 2005. He ordered Katy to report to Montefiore hospital at midnight.

A few hours before, on Halloween night, Katy's family gathered at the Miller home in Creekside. All planned to make the two-hour trip to the hospital: Katy's parents, Roger and Kathy, her four brothers – Bucky, Bryan, twins Jason and Josh – and two of her sisters, Kristy and Ashley. Shelly and Scott drove straight from their home in Cranberry Township, along with their two daughters.

Katy worried about her hair. It was black and soft, and she kept it long and straight. She asked Kristy, who was four years older, to braid it.

"I don't want it to be in my face during the surgery," she told Kristy, who styled it in two rows of French braids.

The family left Creekside in a caravan of three cars. Katy wore her favorite pajamas – yellow cotton pants and matching V-neck top – and terry cloth slippers. Even on the eve of major surgery, with no make-up and a few hours of sleep, Katy looked beautiful. She sat in the back of the car, covered with a blanket.

By the time Roger Miller pulled into the hospital driveway, a light drizzle was falling in the Oakland neighborhood, home to the UPMC medical complex.

The family took over the transplant waiting room on the fifth floor of Montefiore. They rearranged the chairs, placing them together to function as beds. They set up a small table in the middle of the room, where Jason and Josh, the twenty-seven-year-old twins, challenged their brothers and sisters to play poker and Scrabble, Katy's favorite board game. Kristy's co-workers from the National Guard collected money and arranged to deliver subs for lunch and pasta for dinner.

Katy and Shelly checked into the holding area and waited to be wheeled into the OR. They were alone for a short time, two minutes, maybe five, when Katy handed Shelly a note, handwritten on a small white card.

"I'll see you when we get out," Shelly said.

"I love you," Katy replied.

11-1-05

Shelly,

I just wanted to make sure you know how much I truly love you. I know you didn't have to do this for me, but you did, and I will never be able to thank you enough. Mom brought me into this world, but you kept me in it. In more ways than one, you are like a second mother to me. You said that I should only be so lucky to turn out like you and it is true. Hopefully, your cells will make me more domesticated and give me more of a backbone. After we are better, we can have a drinking contest and you will have some competition! It means the world to me that you did this for me and I'll never forget it. I love you with all my heart and soul.

Love,
Katy (AKA Shelly!)

□ ❏ □ ❏ □ ❏ □

The dual surgeries began with Shelly's. All liver-donor surgeries begin this way, donor first, because there must be one final check to ensure the organ is suitable for donation. The donor's surgery also is considered the more high-profile of the two, because the surgeon cuts open a healthy person, putting them at risk for complications, infections and the always-inevitable possibility of death.

Using a Bovie, Marcos opened Shelly's abdomen with a three-way incision that resembles the Mercedes Benz logo – an inverted Y that doctors know as "the chevron." The lines making up the Y are not equal in length. The right one is the longest at about twelve inches. When it reaches the middle of the abdomen, it extends about five inches to the right. At its mid-point, it shoots up toward the chest about three inches.

Marcos lifted Shelly's skin to expose her insides, and ultimately her precious, "sexy" liver. He peeled back her gallbladder, cutting it away from the liver bed. He found the short duct that connects the gallbladder to the common bile duct and inserted a catheter. In preparation for an X-ray, he injected dye that shot up into her common bile duct. The picture showed an outline of Shelly's biliary system, which had to be in top shape for the surgery to proceed.

The X-ray verified what Marcos already knew: Shelly's liver was usable. He picked up a telephone and delivered the final order to the nurses' station: *Get Katy into the operating room. Prepare her for surgery.*

The fifth-floor operating room filled with workers. They had done the surgery many times before, and every one of them knew exactly what to do. Transplant workers don't pussyfoot or think twice about their tasks. They hustle and thrive at the sight of flesh and blood. With the precise choreography of a Broadway musical, one team would take out the right lobe of Shelly's liver, while at the same time, the other tossed out Katy's bag of marbles and prepped her to receive her sister's organ.

Katy lay on a stainless steel gurney, covered with a white sheet. Her braided black hair was covered with a cap, her eyes closed, and her hands on her side, pale and stiff. A nurse placed her in a safe position, making sure she was comfortable and wouldn't strain her muscles or develop pressures sores. She placed a pillow under Katy's knees to relax her legs.

An anesthesiologist inserted a tube down Katy's mouth into her trachea, then plugged it to a ventilator that took over for Katy's breathing. He set up two arterial lines – one in the hand, one in the groin – to measure her heart pressure. He placed major lines in the right internal jugular vein to deliver blood and fluids, and a swan catheter through her heart and into the pulmonary system to track the pressure in her lungs and the strength of her heart. Finally, he inserted a plastic tube known as a bypass cannula into Katy's internal jugular. It would eventually divert blood that would go into her liver and deliver it back to the heart.

There were two surgeons in Katy's room, Ngoc Thai and Kusum Tom. Both were a year out of a transplant fellowship, an academic feat accomplished by only a few hundred surgeons in the United States. Transplant fellows learn to be aggressive and gentle at the same time, asking patients to put their faith in their hands in ways that no other doctor ever does. As they enter the fraternity of transplant surgeons, some recognize their goal is to help patients, not to take risks on their behalf or get caught up in the glory of the profession. Others do not.

Thai and Tom came to know Katy and her family in the weeks leading to the transplant, but the young surgeons had little control over her case. Instead, Marcos ruled. He guided and manipulated every last detail about the surgery. Only he and Starzl could make changes or decisions that would alter the maiden surgery in the protocol. It was almost as if the topic of the protocol was deemed taboo among hospital workers, even if they knew exactly what was going on.

Thai and Tom knew Katy was the first patient in the protocol and were smart enough to understand the implications of her case. They recognized Starzl was transforming the field. He was merging bone marrow transplantation and organ transplantation, which always had been viewed by the immunology community as separate and mutually exclusive.

In the bone marrow procedure, doctors are required to kill the body's entire immune system and replace it with a new one – from the donor. That process becomes tangled in the body of a transplant recipient. The person's immune system is trained to attack the invading donor cells, like a cat that naturally preys on a mouse. Starzl was asking those fully mature cells to act like an immature cell and, in a way, regress so they wouldn't attack the new organ.

It may have been an unprecedented concept, but it came from Starzl, and who was going to question the father of transplantation, an immunologist of the highest degree with worldwide accolades and hundreds of published papers to his name? Certainly no one at UPMC, and certainly not Thai and Tom, who profoundly believed in Starzl's plan. They were eager to participate, to learn from the master and become part of history. And they prepared for the surgery as a quarterback prepares for the Super Bowl, constantly thinking about the case, visualizing the inside of the body, wondering what it would be like on the big day.

A nurse placed sterile blue towels around Katy's bare abdomen, to make sure the area was free of bacteria. Thai grabbed a 4 x 4 gauze sponge, folded it twice and dunked it into a stainless steel bowl filled with betadine. He swabbed the antiseptic on Katy's belly, leaving thick, yellow swirls on her skin.

Thai slid the Bovie just below Katy's ribcage and cut the three incisions that would leave scars on her abdomen for the rest of her life. Unaffected by the smell of burning flesh, Thai lifted Katy's skin. He placed a metal, oval ring over the body and clamped on metal retractors to pull up her ribs.

Just as Tom pulled down Katy's bowels to expose her liver, Marcos took a deep breath in the adjacent OR. He'd done the surgery hundreds of times, but the success of Katy Miller's case had wide-ranging implications. He forced himself to focus on the surgery.

To begin harvesting Shelly's right lobe, Marcos separated the small pieces of tissue that bind the liver to the back of the abdomen. With his glove-covered fingers, he isolated three sections on the liver that supply it with blood on the right side – the hepatic artery, the hepatic vein and the portal vein. He'd wait to cut them off until the end of the surgery. To do otherwise would be disastrous because the liver tissue must be alive and filled with blood when it is cut.

Slicing a liver is not easy. Blood builds up inside it, like water behind a dam, and sticking a knife into it is the equivalent of cutting a bag filled with liquid. Marcos compressed Shelly's liver with his hand and began cutting off its right lobe. It took him nearly four hours to finish. Katy's future – and, coincidentally, his own – was in his hands.

Before sending the liver off to the adjacent operating room, Marcos stuck a tube into the portal vein that feeds into the liver and flushed it with a preservation solution. He put the liver into a bucket of ice and covered it with Saran-wrap and a layer of towels.

Down the hall, the Miller family began to get anxious. They set up a command center in a corner table of the waiting room. They kept a log of everyone who called. They drank coffee, and the kids fell asleep on the floor. They jumped when a nurse or transplant coordinator walked in with an update. When one of them came in, they clustered around to listen.

The removal of the diseased liver is known as a hepatectomy. It is a dangerous, nerve-racking maneuver because surgeons are forced to work near the vena cava. The liver is wrapped around the vena cava, which has led doctors to call it the piggyback part of the surgery. Just a little pinhole can cause significant bleeding.

It took Thai and Tom close to three hours to finish the piggyback. They started by taking down the band of structures that travel from the small bowel to the liver – the portal vein, the hepatic artery and the bile duct. Blood oozed everywhere, as they ruptured tiny blood vessels similar to hemorrhoids that had formed on Katy's sick liver. Blood flowed from every possible crevice. Tom clamped the hepatic vein that empties into the cava and cut out the liver. She threw it into a plastic bag. A lab worker took it to pathology.

Under the microscope, Katy's liver showed signs of evolving cirrhosis, where scar tissue replaces healthy liver tissue. The scarring thwarts the liver's ability to control infections, remove bacteria from the blood, make proteins and dispose of drugs. The inspection of Katy's liver also showed signs of her illness, PSC.

The subsequent pathology report described Katy's liver as having a capsular surface that was "smooth, rubbery to firm, red-gray, with scattered hemorrhagic areas." The liver was 24.5 x 18 x 6.5 centimeters. It weighed a little less than three pounds. The report was essentially the liver's obituary: "The common hepatic duct is dilated exhibiting yellow trabecular mucosa and expressing thick yellow bile and black granular sludge. On dissection, the deep hilum bile ducts are markedly dilated and filled with thick yellow viscous bile and black granular inspissated sludge." It described inflamed bile ducts, edema, lesions and copper accumulation. It wasn't the sexy organ it was supposed to be.

The last part of the transplant marathon required sewing Shelly's right lobe into Katy. Some surgeons say it's the easiest part of the surgery because all they do is sew; others contend it can be challenging because they're putting in half a liver, and how do you know there's enough liver? It would fall on Marcos to do this part of the surgery. It was one of his peculiarities to do this, and it didn't bother the other surgeons. They took a break but remained in the OR, making sure Katy's veins were clean and ready for the new organ.

Using blue, plastic stitches, Marcos sewed Shelly's right hepatic vein to Katy's right hepatic vein. He did it in a running motion, using a single stitch that was looped around both of the blood vessels. He turned to the portal vein and repeated the motion. Once done, he opened the clamped portal vein, releasing blood into the new liver. He did the same with the hepatic vein, which for the first time allowed blood to drain from Katy's new liver into her vena cava, restoring circulation of the liver and bowel.

Using the same kind of sutures, he plugged in the small hepatic artery. This may have been the last leg of the surgery, but represented the riskiest part because of the bile ducts' vulnerability. Without the hepatic artery, the biliary drainage breaks down and the liver is doomed to fail. In the case of Katy, whose bile ducts had been mostly destroyed by her disease, Marcos connected the donor bile duct to her small bowel.

Marcos made sure there was no bleeding anywhere. In a clockwise manner, he checked the different veins, then moved the liver around carefully to check the surrounding tissue for any sign of bleeding – any of the blood that oozed when her sick liver was removed.

Marcos completed the transplant with a plastic surgery closure technique, using absorbable sutures to minimize scarring and help maintain the integrity of Katy's young body. Within twenty minutes, Katy was on her way to the intensive care unit.

Nurses wheeled her into the hallway, and her family stampeded out of the waiting room. They cried as they watched her pass, tubes stuck in her mouth, eyes still closed, hair still neatly braided.

□ ◻ □ ◻ □ ◻ □

The Miller family stood at attention as the gurneys poked out of the large metal doors. First Shelly, then Katy. Shelly was awake but groggy, and everyone felt relieved to see her open eyes. Scott touched her hand as she went by. Katy was not awake. Her eyes were taped shut, and she didn't seem to be breathing on her own. For her parents, brothers and sisters, the sight of Katy so helpless and vulnerable jolted them into reality. Katy was in serious condition, and her recovery could be long and tenuous. Her mother and sisters cried. The men also struggled to contain the tears.

The transplant intensive care unit at Montefiore has two long wings, with rooms that have large windows so nurses have a direct line of sight. The unit boasted one of the country's top transplant teams. UPMC hired the best surgeons and the best supporting staff. There were specially trained anesthesiologists, pathologists and psychiatrists. All patients were assisted by a transplant coordinator – a registered nurse who acts almost as an air traffic controller at a busy airport. Instead of tracking flights in the sky and watching a Doppler radar, a transplant coordinator tracks blood tests, CT scans and clinic appointments.

The intensive care unit may have been in a 100-year-old building, but administrators outfitted it with sophisticated monitoring systems and the latest ventilators, infusion pumps and emergency resuscitation equipment.

Katy recovered in a room two doors down from her sister's. The sisters couldn't see each other. Katy didn't know where Shelly was, and Shelly didn't know where Katy was. The family took turns visiting their rooms, and nurses joked about building a special waiting room for them.

Nurses extubated Katy the day after the surgery. The narcotics injected into her veins played cruel games with her mind. She woke up agitated and confused. She saw spiders and bugs everywhere in her hospital room – on the floor, on her night stand, on her bed. Katy screamed at the top of her lungs: "Get the spiders off me!"

The screams shook the intensive care unit and traveled all the way down to Shelly's room, two doors down. Shelly called for a nurse and asked what was happening.

"What's wrong with my sister? Take me to see her," Shelly ordered.

Across the hall, she found Katy on her bed, sweat on her forehead, still rattled and almost shaking.

They had her strapped down, but she remained agitated, as if she wanted to run out of the hospital.

"Take the spiders off me!" she screamed.

"Katy, calm down," Shelly said.

The hallucinations Katy experienced were a common side effect of the painkillers. While Katy saw spiders and bugs, some patients are tormented by disturbing visions of long-dead relatives or religious figures.

Nurses warned Katy's family not to massage her legs or feet – a favorite pleasure – because it could break off a blood clot. Kathy's mother took the warning seriously and forbid her other children to break the rule. Jason didn't listen.

"Can you rub my legs?" Katy said.

"Of course," Jason replied. He was happy to do something for his sister.

Over the next days in ICU, relatives brought bags of food to feed the family. There were too many of them, and eating out near the hospital became too expensive. Katy's Aunt Linda delivered trays of stuffed cabbage, pots of home-made chili and her famous Gob cake, a family favorite with icing on the inside instead of outside.

Kristy wheeled a hair wash station into the room to clean Katy's hair.

She vigorously scrubbed her sister's scalp. She dried it and often braided it, if only to pass time.

"Mom, tickle my forehead," Katy said. Kathy stood by her daughter's side and placed her fingers above Katy's eyes, gently rubbing her eyebrows.

The gentle touch of her mother's hand was like a magic pill that sometimes took away the pain. Yet, often the pain prevailed, and Katy felt as if her stomach was being ripped open. She pressed a pillow against her stomach when she needed to cough. She agonized even more when she heard Shelly was still hurting.

"I wish they could take all of Shelly's pain and give it to me," she told Shelly's husband, Scott.

A week after the transplant, Katy underwent a Doppler sonogram of her new liver. The medical records gave a promising outlook: *The right lobe transplant is sonographically normal. No intra or extrahepatic biliary ductal dilation is seen and there are no perihepatic fluid collections.*

After eight days in the ICU, typical for a liver transplant recipient, Katy became in tune with her body and the effects of major surgery and the drugs that followed. She knew to protest if she was given oxycodone and to approve when the painkiller of choice was dilaudid.

"Give me dilaudid. It doesn't freak me out," she told the nurse.

Marcos discharged her on November 10, nine days after the transplant. The two-page summary showed the live-donor liver transplant on Katy Miller, a nineteen-year-old Caucasian female, and the donor operation of her thirty-three-year-old sister, had been conducted without incident. Katy was leaving the hospital on a regular diet that she tolerated well, stable vital signs, improved liver function tests and controlled pain. She also was leaving with a list of nine medications, numbered alongside their dosage.

1. Prograf 1.5 mg p.o. twice a day

2. *Aspirin 81 mg p.o. q. a.m.*

3. *Actigall 300 mg p.o. 3 times a day*

4. *Protonix 40 mg p.o. q. daily*

5. *Nystatin 5 ml swish and swallow p.o. 4 times a day*

6. *Acyclovir 200 mg p.o. twice a day*

7. *Bactrium SS 1 tablet p.o. every Monday, Wednesday and Friday*

8. *Magnesium gluconate 1500 mg p.o. 3 times a day*

9. *Darvocet-N 100 one tablet p.o. every six hours p.r.n. pain for 2 weeks*

It was no mistake that the number one drug was Prograf, the nasty anti-rejection medicine that would stop Katy's immune system from ambushing her brand new liver. Marcos and Starzl vowed that Katy wouldn't have to take the drugs for long.

Katy left the hospital confident that her doctors had told her the truth.

6

Medical icon

Few birthday parties feature pipe organ music, but Thomas Starzl's eightieth would have to be different. Starzl was a devoted fan of Mozart, and administrators at the University of Pittsburgh envisioned a special tribute featuring music from the famous composer. What better way to honor the father of organ transplantation than with an organ version of a Mozart masterpiece?

The university chancellor asked renowned organist and professor Robert Sutherland Lord to create an organ rendition of Don Giovanni, one of Mozart's most popular operas.

The result was cleverly titled "Mozart Transplantation for Organ" and recorded by Sutherland at Heinz Memorial Chapel, famous for its acoustics and stunning stained-glass. Sutherland's seven-minute creation combined a folk-like duet, "La ci darem la mano," with music by a friend of Mozart's, Franz Joseph Haydn, that was used as the university's alma mater.

Starzl loved it. He smiled broadly as he listened to the powerful sounds of the organ and recognized the work of his idol. He'd first talked publicly about his love of Mozart at the International Organ Transplant Forum in 1987.

"How much more complete might the world have been if Mozart had been treated with renal transplantation instead of dying of glomerulo-nephritis at the age of thirty-five?" Starzl said.

More than 400 guests packed the historic Connolly ballroom on the first floor of Alumni Hall in Oakland, six blocks from the hospital where Starzl once ruled the operating rooms.

The birthday festivities, barely four months after Katy's liver transplant, would last two days and include a scientific symposium titled, "Transplant Tolerance: The challenges ahead." It was an oversized celebration, fitting for a man with a big ego.

During his glory days in 1985, Starzl bragged to a reporter from *The Pittsburgh Press* that foreign patients came to Pittsburgh because of the transplant program's prominence.

"They come because they know we can do things here that no one, anywhere else in the world, can do," he said.

He had a right to brag. In the late 1980s, Starzl and his team performed more than 500 liver transplants a year, more than any other center in the United States. Starzl was the transplant king, once traveling from Pittsburgh to Texas, where he helped Baylor University Medical Center establish its transplant program by performing back-to-back liver transplants on the same day.

Starzl looked dapper in a smart, light-brown suit and never strayed too far from his second wife, Joy, who wore a colorful striped suit. The surgeon didn't look his age. He was a vigorous octogenarian, trim and with a full head of gray hair. He shook hands with the biggest names in transplantation, who flew in to offer their well-wishes: Kathryn Wood of Oxford University, an expert in the field of tolerance and immunology; Sir Roy Calne of the University of Cambridge, knighted for his achievements in organ transplantation and proving the effectiveness of the anti-rejection drug cyclosporine; Dr. Nancy Ascher, chair of surgery at the University of California; Dr. Chris Larsen, surgery chief at Emory University and known for his work in developing new immunologic drugs.

Standing under one of several massive chandeliers, Starzl beamed as he greeted and hugged more than one hundred former transplant fellows he had mentored. One by one, they came to pay their respects and the often long-winded Starzl worried he wouldn't have time to talk to all of them. Starzl had trained almost every transplant surgeon in the country, connecting Pittsburgh to the more than a hundred transplant centers in the nation.

Among those snapping pictures next to Starzl was Katy Miller. He placed his arm around Katy's back and pulled her against him, their shoulders touching as Katy smiled. A few months before, Katy's beautiful dark eyes and soft black hair captivated Starzl when they met for the first time in a room at Montefiore hospital. Katy had been undergoing tests and screenings required before the operation; Starzl walked in and startled her as she read a book.

"Hello," she said, not sure of who he was. She'd heard about him but didn't know what he looked like.

"Tom Starzl," he said.

She suddenly straightened up, the way children do when the principal shows up in the classroom. She closed her book and quickly ran her hands through her hair.

"Nice to meet you, Dr. Starzl," she said. "I've heard a lot about you."

"They told me you were pretty, but they didn't tell me you were beautiful," Starzl said, causing her to blush.

Marcos walked into the Connolly ballroom alone, wearing a bright orange tie, with a ready smile and tousled hair. He greeted his young patient with a warm embrace. A few days before the party, Marcos had asked Katy, who was several weeks away from turning twenty, what she planned to wear to the event.

"Do you know what kind of dress you need to wear to this type of party?" Marcos asked.

"No. I think I might just wear some shorty shorts," Katy snapped, annoyed that Marcos would consider her so unsophisticated. What did Marcos possibly think she would wear?

Katy wore an elegant white pant suit and a black blouse. She turned eyes with her youth and wide smile, followed closely by her mother and sister, Shelly.

Starzl invited Katy and her family to a meeting room off the ballroom where guests ate ice cream in honor of Starzl's hometown of LeMars, Iowa, known as the "Ice Cream Capital of the World." Guests prepared sundaes and banana splits, and Katy playfully squirmed when she dripped ice cream on someone's shoe.

A smitten Starzl introduced Katy to the University of Pittsburgh chancellor, the dean of the medical school and Art Rooney II, president of the Pittsburgh Steelers. He spoke with a steady voice and was mindful to mention why she was attending the party.

Dr. Thomas Starzl was a proud man. The young woman before him, he explained, was the first of 10 patients in an ambitious trial of an immunosuppressive drug protocol at the university. Katy had just received a liver transplant four months ago, and her prognosis was excellent, he told some guests at the party. Starzl fussed over Katy the way a grandfather shows off a first grandchild. He made sure to praise Shelly and her decision to put herself through major surgery for Katy's sake. The sisters and their mother felt welcome and special, even among people so high up in the medical hierarchy.

"Doesn't she look marvelous?" Starzl was overheard saying to one of the guests.

Starzl thrived in the spotlight. He'd turned on the charm many times before, in front of TV cameras and on the cover of magazines. He worked the ballroom for a few hours, trying not to spend too much time with someone so he wouldn't offend those who were waiting to get up close. One of the guests was Betty Baird, one of Starzl's first patients at the University of Colorado in Denver.

Betty sat at a table not far from Katy, but the two never had a chance to talk. Unbeknownst to Katy, Betty was one of a handful of transplant recipients in the world living without taking anti-rejection medicine.

Betty was a twenty-two-year-old newlywed when she received a badly needed liver on December 1, 1979, in a procedure that was barely in its infancy and considered anything but standard.

Doctors in her hometown of Hopwood, Pennsylvania, had given her a month to live. They didn't know what was wrong with her. When she ate anything salty or high in sodium, it caused fluid buildup and excessive swelling. No one could give her a straight answer, other than to tell Betty that her liver was nearly destroyed and beyond repair. Her doctor read about the transplant surgery in a medical journal and proposed it as a solution of last resort.

Her husband convinced her to go for it. Otherwise, he was certain she would die. Betty traveled to Denver, leaving her husband behind. No one in her family could afford to make the trip. To make her feel better, nurses put a Christmas tree in her hospital room. Starzl, who was fifty-three at the time, performed the liver transplant. The organ came from a twenty-one-year-old woman who'd died in a car crash. The miraculous surgery saved Betty's life.

Two years later, after giving birth to her daughter, Lori, Betty began to question the logic of taking so much immunosuppression. The daily doses of prednisone and imuran were causing extreme changes in her mood, and she didn't like it.

"The anti-rejection medicine makes you go happy one minute, sad the next," she told me later. "The emotions were too up and down."

In a moment of desperation, Betty flushed the pills down the toilet. "I just decided it had to stop," she said. "I was young and stupid. I wasn't thinking what it could do to me."

"You'll die without the drugs," someone told her.

Without the medicine, doctors had warned she would begin rejecting her liver. That was in August 1981. Thirty years later, Betty had never experienced a symptom of rejection. And all the while, she avoided the nasty complications that tend to come with the drugs.

Betty told me she had to survive to take care of her daughter. When she had a bad day, she tried to think of how sick she had been and how close she was to leaving her daughter without a mom. She told me about taking a job as a nursing assistant in her local hospital. She became overly stressed and one day left work in the middle of her shift, breathing heavily with an overabundance of adrenaline. Once home, she rummaged through the drawers in her dresser. Tucked in one of them was a folded piece of paper. She opened it and read it. It was a letter that Lori, her daughter, had written to Starzl. *Thank you for saving my mother's life.* Betty cried as she read. She thought about her daughter writing a thank-you, not knowing what else to do to show her gratitude. *You can give the mailman a box of cookies, but what do you give a man who saved your life?*

"God didn't save me to sit on my butt the rest of my life," she said. "Life is a chance. You have to take chances."

Betty hugged Starzl tightly at the birthday party, a reaction Starzl had come to expect from former patients. She spoke to him for a few minutes before he had to walk away to give a welcoming speech. She sat next to Bob Phillips, who'd come from Virginia with his niece despite having just turned eighty years old four months before.

"I'm not going to refuse any invitation," Phillips said.

Phillips in 2004 had been recognized as the oldest living organ transplant recipient. His kidney transplant surgery had been done by Starzl on January 30, 1963, at the University of Colorado. Phillips was living in Virginia at the time, his kidneys destroyed and living only because of dialysis. Doctors had told him he had days to live.

His younger sister, Ruth, had seen a story in the newspaper about Starzl's work in Denver. She called the hospital, asking if she could donate one of her kidneys.

Phillips stayed in Denver for three years after the surgery, working for Starzl by doing odd jobs and speaking to patients and families about his experience with transplantation.

"I idolize Dr. Starzl," Phillips said.

Bob Phillips was a survivor in a medical world filled with chances, risks – and death. Thomas Starzl had saved him in exactly the same way he had saved Katy. Starzl could now celebrate his triumphs – giving life and cheating death.

If Starzl was so determined to save lives – the Betty Bairds, the Bob Phillips and the Katy Millers of the world – it was because death had tricked him countless times during his life. In many ways, it was as if Starzl was obsessed with death.

His first encounter with death hurt the most because it was his mother, Anna. She had breast cancer and became sick during Starzl's final days at Westminster College in Fulton, Missouri. She couldn't attend her son's graduation, and he had to rush home immediately after getting his diploma. The young Starzl had been instructed to help with his mother's care. If she became restless or complained of pain, he'd been told to give her an injection of morphine in her buttock or hip. In those days, morphine didn't come readily prepared the way it is today. Starzl had to dissolve a tablet in a tablespoon of tap water and draw it into a syringe. When his mother told him she was suffocating, he rushed to the kitchen to prepare the injection. His anxiety overwhelmed him, and he dropped the spoon on the floor. He tried a second time but by the time he reached his mother, she was nearly gone. He blamed himself for her death for years.

Then there were the dogs – the ones he carefully sliced open in Miami during his medical training. More than fifty years later, when I asked Starzl about the dogs, he refused to talk about it.

"Talk to me about the dogs and the early experiments," I asked him.

"I'm not going to talk about that," he said.

"Why?"

"I have nightmares about it."

The images of the hopeless dogs – the animals that began the revolution to organ transplantation – had stayed in Starzl's mind all these years. I was stunned. Yet in more ways than one, it helped explain his love of dogs in his later years. After his retirement from the operating room, he could be seen walking in the heart of the Oakland university district, his hand tightly wrapped around several dog chains. All five of them were female.

"They are much gentler dogs," he told me.

Starzl sounded both proud and worried when he told me about his new puppy, a Golden Retriever he had picked up at a breeder an hour north of Pittsburgh. He'd driven himself to get the puppy on a windy day, traveling on Route 28 – the same highway that led to Katy Miller's house in Creekside.

"She's very bright," he told me when the puppy was about eight weeks old. "But she has trouble holding her urine."

Starzl had named the puppy Chooloo, after a stray mutt named Koochooloo in the bestselling novel "Cutting for Stone," a book he had just finished reading that delves into the power and responsibility of being a doctor. Starzl shortened the name because he found Koochooloo too cumbersome. In the novel, by Abraham Verghese, Koochooloo avoids people after desperately watching workers in a mission clinic asphyxiate her puppies in a plastic bag. There was no doubt in my mind that the puppies' fate must have resonated with Starzl and taken him back to his days in a dark Miami garage.

"I'm off today," Starzl told me, an unusual statement coming from someone his age. "I need to stay home and make sure she learns how to do this."

It turned out Chooloo had been able to hold herself and do her business at the right time, but when Starzl picked her up to congratulate her, she started to leak.

"She was too excited," he said, explaining the amount of urine on the floor the way doctors measure medicine. "She let go about ten or fifteen cc's of urine."

"So how many dogs do you have now?" I asked.

"Six," he said. "But you know Ophelia is in her last days."

Ophelia, a half-collie he found on the doorstep of his house, had been Starzl's constant companion over the years. She accompanied him on walks and slept at his feet in the office. She went with him to lunch and often rode with him in his car. She even appeared with her master on the cover of Pittsburgh magazine in 2001.

"She's been having trouble getting around," he told me matter of factly. "She had an ear stroke six months ago."

Starzl didn't exactly say it, but I could tell Chooloo's presence could help him tolerate the pain that Ophelia's imminent death would bring. Death had surrounded him during his lifetime, but how could it not?

The gruesome and bloody nature of organ transplantation made it inevitable that Starzl's career would involve deaths – and many of them. Some deaths had been unexpected, others perhaps necessary. Starzl grieved every single one of them.

During his surgical training, he dreaded going to the morgue at Jackson Memorial in Miami, where he faced dozens of corpses – all potential blood vessel donors. In his memoir, he described the donors as "a parade of sorrow: drowned children; raped and murdered women; blond, suntanned muscle-builders with neat bullet holes in their heads; and victims of automobile accidents."

In his early days in medicine – in Miami, and later in Chicago and Denver – surgeries were never easy because of the prospect of death. He feared that he wouldn't be able to help the hopeful patients who came to him to be fixed. The surgeries didn't come easy, and Starzl agonized right up to their very beginning. In the days leading up to the surgery, he studied books and notes and memorized every single detail of the operation.

In his early surgical training, he considered not replacing the liver with a new one, but instead adding a second liver to the human body. He figured out this could be much easier because it would not require the technically demanding operation to remove the diseased liver.

Much to Starzl's dismay, his first attempt at a human liver transplant on March 1, 1963, ended in misfortune. The patient was a three-year-old boy named Bennie Solis. The boy bled to death because his blood would not clot. Surgeons stayed in the operating room for hours, silent. Some wept. They never forgot Bennie.

When Starzl arrived in Pittsburgh in December 1980, there were deaths there, too. The first four liver transplant patients at then Presbyterian University Hospital died. But it was the case of a girl named Stormie Jones that rattled Starzl the most.

Stormie was a freckle-faced, six-year-old from Ft. Worth, Texas, who had been born with a genetic condition that put her cholesterol level at ten times higher than normal. She'd led an ordinary childhood until her mother, Lois Purcell, found her skin covered with tiny bumps that resembled warts. They were on her elbows, knuckles, knees and toes. The bumps were deposits of cholesterol that also were blocking her arteries. The little girl suffered a heart attack in October 1983. Doctors were stumped. They tried two bypass surgeries but they didn't work.

It was a problem with her liver – the organ that was supposed to remove the bad cholesterol, or LDL, from the walls of her blood vessels. The answer would be a liver transplant, but Stormie's heart was so weak from her illness that doctors didn't think she could survive the operation. They chose to give her not just a liver, but also a new heart.

On Valentine's Day 1984, Stormie became the world's first recipient of a simultaneous heart-liver transplant. The fifteen-hour surgery performed by Starzl made headlines around the world. Stormie received her new organs from a four-year-old girl in New York who had died in a traffic accident. The transplant was a success, and Stormie went back to her hometown. She was able to eat hamburgers and hot dogs, although doctors restricted her diet to vegetables and skim milk. Hepatitis, however, eventually threatened to destroy her liver. Stormie returned to Pittsburgh in February 1990 and underwent a second liver transplant. Early that November, she was back at the hospital, complaining of flu-like symptoms – a sore throat, low-grade fever and dehydration. She died November 11 after rejecting her heart. Doctors found the rejection, so long after the transplant, extremely unusual.

Starzl was shocked. It was time to quit. He couldn't see himself becoming emotionally attached to more patients only to lose them without warning. He was emotionally drained. He announced his retirement. It was November 1990.

"When you lose a patient like that, it's awful," he said at the time, when he was sixty-four.

He didn't exactly retire. He was a slave to his own mind and talent. His days in the operating room may have been over, but he had much more to accomplish. What good was cutting up a person, sewing in an organ and closing them back up if there was a battalion of immune system cells ready to attack the new organ? It was a question that haunted him from the very beginning of the field, when he was slicing up dogs in Colorado in the fall of 1963. In those days, doing liver transplants on dogs, Starzl discovered it was possible to stop anti-rejection treatment three or four months after the surgery without prompting the animals to reject their new organs. He called it a drug-free state in which the animals' immune system surrendered against the new organ. "You can stay, we won't harm you," the immune system seemed to say, acting contrary to the way it was supposed to behave. It's possible that Starzl's obsession with organ rejection was born in those days. There had to be a way to control rejection, whether it was a kidney or liver. He was sure of that. How to do it would be the next step. If anyone could figure that out, he wanted to be the one. And who cared if he had retired? In many ways, he was the perfect man to do it. He had thrown so many Hail Marys and completed so many of them, it made sense for him to chase this dream.

Starzl dedicated his time to scrutinize chimerism. It was a make-or-break challenge. That's what led him to Katy and the ambitious plan to wean her off immunosuppression. He wasn't content with fifty-year-old achievements. He longed to walk off the international platform with one thunderous final act to cement his legacy as a master of 20th century medicine.

Starzl could have just waltzed into retirement. All signs pointed to a triumphant exit. UPMC in 1994 renamed its program as the Thomas E. Starzl Transplantation Institute. In 2006, it also named a nine-story biomedical science tower after Starzl, just across the street from a hall named after polio pioneer Jonas Salk. Starzl enjoyed the attention that came with these honors: fancy dinners with scholars and alumni and effusive speeches about his greatness.

Just a month before the 80th birthday party, accolades arrived from President George W. Bush. The 43rd president granted Starzl one of the nation's highest honors, the National Medal of Science. The surgeon wore

Pittsburgh colors to the White House ceremony – a black and gold necktie. As Bush put the medal on his neck, Starzl jokingly whispered that the Steelers, brand-new Super Bowl champions, would surely visit the White House in the coming weeks.

Top leaders from the medical center watched from the audience, including Jeffrey Romoff and Dr. Timothy Billiar, the chief of surgery. Marcos was there, too.

Marcos' presence at the White House – and at the birthday celebration – seemed odd. He and Starzl had never gotten along, even though Starzl approved of his hiring. Starzl once deadpanned that he'd never been to Marcos' home for dinner, and Starzl had never invited Marcos to his own house. But they tolerated each other, profoundly aware that they needed each other to survive. Marcos needed Starzl's name to build his reputation. And Starzl needed Marcos to help write the last chapter of his storied career.

Starzl would be the mastermind behind the ambitious protocol to treat liver transplant recipients such as Katy. Marcos would be the quarterback, doing the surgeries, caring for the patients and calling the shots based on their recovery.

Marcos was perfect for the part. He was young and eager to learn, with an appetite for power and fame. His good looks worked to his advantage. He could seduce women – and potential transplant candidates – with his *GQ* appearance, debonair approach and charismatic eyes. Where Starzl was all brain, Marcos had sex appeal.

The disparity troubled Starzl but he was smart enough to keep any thoughts to himself. He heard about Marcos' Casanova reputation but chose to keep his opinion to himself. Not that he would forget; Starzl was known for his legendary memory. At the height of his career, he wrote a scientific paper every week and remembered with exact precision the names of all journal publications, down to the volume and page numbers.

"Terry, get me the Helsinki paper," he would shout to his assistant, Terry Mangan. There was no need to give her a year or a citation. She knew exactly which paper he meant.

Starzl also remembered the name and hometown of every patient. He didn't just perform a transplant surgery and walk out; he spent time with each patient and asked questions about families, jobs, and schools. He wanted to know everything and gave patients the most precious commodity in medicine – time. Starzl stayed up twenty-four hours doing surgeries, only to finish up and walk to the surgical floors to visit his patients. The fellows couldn't keep up with his energy. He often slept in his office. Even when he went home, he picked up the phone and called the nurses to ask about his patients.

While some people who worked with him say Starzl had a propensity to be conceited, some thought he came across as unassuming. Terri Caponi, a nurse who later became a transplant coordinator, recalled seeing him for the first time in the early 1980s. Starzl wore a black turtleneck and a red windbreaker as he stood at a nurses' station.

"Who's the fisherman?" Caponi asked one of her fellow nurses.

"Shut up Terri. That's Starzl," her colleague replied.

"No way. That's Starzl?"

❑ ❑ ❑ ❑ ❑ ❑ ❑

The first time I met Starzl in January 2006, he looked almost like a fisherman. He was wearing a bright orange coat, holding a black umbrella, and beads of rain ran across his forehead. I'd been waiting for him nearly 30 minutes in his office, across the street from Children's Hospital of Pittsburgh, surrounded by stacks of books, rusted filing cabinets and walls with pictures of his glory days as Pittsburgh's star transplant surgeon. The scent of dog hair lingered in the air.

I was interviewing him for a story about the National Medal of Science, clearly a happy occasion, but Starzl seemed highly annoyed when he walked in. His ever-present dogs followed him, including then eight-year-old Ophelia. Here he was, the father of organ transplantation, the man who performed the first successful human liver transplant, and he just seemed like a retired grandfather preoccupied with his pets.

"We should probably hustle," said Starzl, noting that he was being interviewed by his hometown newspaper in LeMars, Iowa, a few hours later. "I am just about being exploited."

In our first few minutes together, I found him dry and cerebral. He gave me long-winded answers about his legacy and jumped from one subject to another, with fast words that made it hard to understand. He was cynical when I asked about his legacy. He told me his achievements were anything but sensational because they stretched across more than four decades.

"When things develop like that, it's a little bit like watching grass grow," he told me. "All of a sudden it's grown, and it doesn't seem like anything very dramatic."

When the subject turned to matters other than medicine and organ transplantation, he loosened up. He asked where I was from, and when I told him Puerto Rico, he told me about a man who once approached him when he was at a beach on the island. The man asked Starzl if he was wearing a toupee. Starzl said no, but the man reached to Starzl's hair and pulled it, trying to catch him in a lie.

A month later, in February 2006, I saw him again in Washington, D.C., where he was about to get the National Medal of Science. I watched from an area cordoned off for journalists where I could see other award recipients such as filmmaker George Lucas, creator of *Star Wars* and *Indiana Jones*, who was receiving the National Medal of Science and Technology. Starzl and I had our photograph taken outside the White House, and he introduced me to his wife, Joy, and his grandson, Ravi.

Starzl and I clicked. He seemed to like me, and I liked the way he reminded me of my grandfather, Carlos, who, like Starzl, had deep respect for journalists. Starzl and I spoke occasionally, and I always seemed to catch him when he was back from a trip abroad. Once, fresh from a trip to London, he spoke about watching the French movie *I've Loved You For So Long* with English actress Kristin Scott Thomas. He found the movie, about a woman released from prison after a fifteen-year sentence, stunning and deeply moving. But he didn't stop there. He lectured me about the golden age of cinema and lamented the commercialization of movies.

One other time, he started talking about having an "in-flight complication" when he experienced a deep venous thrombosis in his left leg. He told me about going on the blood thinner Heparin, but not before warning me that he was breaking federal privacy rules by revealing details of his own health. I had to hold myself from laughing. Within minutes, he'd started talking about the economic crisis in the United States, sharing his belief that "it looks more like a depression than a recession." Starzl had an opinion about everything.

One cold winter morning in 2010, we met for lunch. I wanted to talk to him about writing a book about Katy. We had talked about Katy many times over the past year, and I was eager to give him an update. "I'd love to see you," he had told me a few days before when I reached him on his cell phone.

Panera, a busy sandwich joint on Pitt's campus was a Starzl favorite, perhaps because it put him closer to his days as a star surgeon two decades earlier. The place buzzes with students and professors, some of them alone with their laptops, others engaged in lively study-group discussions. Starzl preferred a closed-off room with glass walls in the back corner, ideal for a man who treasured privacy.

Starzl placed the plastic lunch tray on the table and loosened the Burberry scarf around his neck. On the tray was a salad, a grilled turkey sandwich and an apple. He looked sharp in a smart, light-colored suit and heavy, mustard-colored boots.

When I told him I liked his scarf, he said his wife gave it to him. "Do you know the right way to wear it?" he asked. I told him I did, but he showed me how to tie it anyway, folding it in half and making a loop in which he then inserted the other end. That was the Starzl way, never to be outdone or outsmarted, even if it was a trivial fashion issue. A few weeks before, when we talked at a reception for Carnegie Science Award recipients, he chastised me for wearing brown shoes with a blue suit.

This time around, as I watched him pick off the edges of his sandwich, there was little chastising, but a gentle preaching. I had spoken not two sentences about my book project when he jumped in to talk about his own publishing experience. In 1992, he published *The Puzzle People*, a memoir printed by the University of Pittsburgh Press. He had no book agent and placed calls on his own to several big-name publishers. However interested, the editors demanded too much, and Starzl opted to write the book on his own, in his own way. No one was going to tell him how to do it, he told me.

Yet here he was, about to tell me that my book would not accomplish anything because it wouldn't change the outcome.

"It's all over," he said.

Starzl's words, stinging yet candid, moved me in an unexpected way. Oddly, they persuaded me not to let go of the project and embrace it with passion I never knew I had. The more he spoke about roadblocks and impossibilities, the more I wanted to get it done. I took a sip of my coffee, cold after two hours of intense conversation, and told Starzl so.

"It's not going to change what happened," he said.

Our conversation grew awkward and strained. Starzl tried to change the subject and fidgeted with his cardboard coffee cup. I sensed he would rather be talking about football than liver transplants. But I knew the man sitting before me cared deeply about Katy.

"Have you talked to the Miller family?" he said.

"Of course, I have, Dr. Starzl," I said. "They are very supportive of this project."

I told Starzl that I spoke to Katy's mom regularly, sometimes two or three times a week, and sometimes I couldn't stop her from talking. She was a reporter's dream, willing to answer the same question over and over. She was eager for me to tell her daughter's story.

"You have to be careful," he said. "You don't want to come across like you are using the family just to get a book published."

I valued Starzl's words. Not because of who he was, but because there was something about the way he spoke – the magnitude of words almost too large for this world – that nearly hypnotized me.

"I better get going," he told me that February morning.

He carried his plastic tray to the trash can and held on to his cup of coffee. We walked out of the restaurant together, along snow-covered Fifth Avenue. Dirty slush splashed on his dress pants. Starzl stopped and looked me straight in the eyes. I thought he was going to lecture me, but he did not.

"You have a good heart," he said. "You'll get the book done."

I watched him go across the street and thought about the first time I met him – the beads of rain on his forehead, the look of a fisherman. It struck me that I had looked at his hands during lunch, and they reminded me of the hands of a fisherman. They were strong, sturdy and calloused – the hands used to fillet a snapper or a mackerel. Only Starzl's hands had once sliced open humans to sew in new organs.

7

Yellow all over

Ashley noticed it first. She looked at Katy's eyes and did a double take. They were yellow.

It was a peculiar shade of yellow, too, like an old newspaper that's starting to fade. It was subtle, but it didn't look right. Ashley said nothing, even though she wanted to look at Katy's eyes again. *Is it my imagination or just a reflection of the sun?*

The two sisters had spent the morning shopping for new outfits at the mall in Indiana and were headed back to Creekside. Katy turned up the music as they drove back home. Ashley stole a quick glance at Katy's eyes. No doubt, they were yellow.

Ashley was 16 and had watched her sister's battle with PSC from a distance, not because she didn't care but because it was hard to understand. Ashley was struck by the look in Katy's eyes. The yellow color made them mysterious, as if they were hiding something.

As soon as they got home, Ashley pulled her mother aside.

"Her eyes look yellow, Mom," she whispered.

"I know, I noticed, too," Kathy Miller told the youngest of her eight children.

The yellow in Katy's eyes was, in the simplest terms, not a good sign. Medically, it meant that her bilirubin levels were high. Bilirubin is a brownish yellow substance in bile, which is made by the liver to help digest fat. Bilirubin is produced when the liver breaks down old red blood cells. Most of it is waste that winds up being expelled through the bile duct into the small intestine, then exits the body in the stool.

Bilirubin can be stubborn. Maternity wards have special lights to treat high bilirubin in jaundiced newborns because too much of it can damage their brains. Bile can build up in the bile ducts that carry it from the liver, much like fatty materials build up in the inner lining of arteries and cause strokes and heart attacks.

In a liver transplant, the lack of blood supply can cause scar tissue to build up inside the tiny bile ducts. The blockage causes the yellowish bilirubin to accumulate in the blood.

The excess bilirubin changes the color of skin and the whites of the eyes. In patients with liver disease, it is a cruel reminder of what's happening inside their bodies. Many of them are bewildered by the irony – yellow is supposed to be the color of hope and wisdom.

There are various degrees of yellow, some more noticeable than others. Some people look like they have a slight sun tan. The most acute of liver problems cause so much back-up of bilirubin that skin turns the color of a canary.

When a person begins to turn yellow, it portends one of two

problems: a plumbing issue within the bile duct or a malfunction of the liver that prevents it from converting bile into a soluble form that can be excreted in urine. Surgeons don't know why this happens, but they know that when bile backs up, it can create infections and cirrhosis – a disease many associate with alcoholism that often is a precursor to a liver transplant.

It was fall 2006, when leaves were changing color and the air was cooler. As Katy approached the first anniversary of her transplant, her skin began to itch. She scratched her legs, arms, thighs, even the top of her feet. Initially, she suspected mosquito bites because she'd been spending time outside in the back of her house, which is surrounded by trees and grass. An in-ground pool also attracted insects.

But the itching never seemed to stop. Katy scratched hard with her long finger nails, tearing her skin until she drew blood. It's like it's itching *inside* my skin, she'd tell her mother. It hurt so much she cried.

Kathy called Terri, Katy's transplant coordinator at UPMC. She spoke to Terri every day, sometimes two or three times. Terri's job was to keep an eye on Katy, the way an FBI agent keeps an eye on a suspected terrorist.

"What do you think it is?" Kathy said.

"She has to come in," Terri told her. "No need to worry. We'll figure it out."

Eight months earlier, Marcos had begun weaning Katy off the Prograf. She initially took two capsules of the drug every day. Two months after the surgery, the dose was cut to once a day. Three months later, it went down to every other day.

Marcos now ordered a liver function panel to measure blood levels of total protein, albumin, bilirubin and liver enzymes. The elevated numbers merely confirmed what any good doctor would have suspected from seeing Katy's yellow skin and eyes: her liver was clearly showing signs of malfunction. Something was wrong. A liver biopsy followed. Katy would be sedated, the skin under her belly numbed so that an interventional radiologist could insert a needle under her ribcage. The goal: to rip out a tiny piece of her liver no bigger than a peanut.

According to her medical records, the liver biopsy "showed evidence of a mild rejection reaction." Over a period of several months, the records said, biopsies showed "increasingly severe changes of biliary tract obstruction/structuring. Biliary strictures were eventually documented cholangiographically and portal hypertension developed."

Katy looked at herself in the mirror with a mixture of sadness and confusion. She was supposed to be at the peak of her beauty and confidence, getting close to her 21st birthday, not feeling bloated and weak. A doctor prescribed Benadryl; Katy slathered herself with the lotion. Questions haunted her as she dug into her skin. *Am I always going to be yellow? Will I ever get better? Will I ever be normal?*

Katy's body was rebelling. The tiny bile ducts were so narrowed that bile was building up inside them at a fast pace. Doctors refer to the problem as biliary strictures. They are uncommon, but often unavoidable. They were slowly destroying Katy's bile duct system.

Katy's belly grew bigger, the victim of ascites, a fluid buildup dreaded by liver disease patients. The fluid was lodging in a membrane called the peritoneum. The membrane has two layers, one lining the abdominal wall and another that wraps organs like the liver, stomach and intestines. The fluid, usually present in very small quantities, serves as a lubricant that essentially allows the organs to glide over one another. As more fluid collected in her abdomen, Katy became increasingly bloated. She was in pain, uncomfortable and didn't want to eat.

The rapid decline in Katy's health bewildered her entire family. Like everyone else, Kathy believed Katy's transplant had saved her daughter. She'd been amazed by Katy's resilience and her daughter's positive attitude. Katy had vowed to be normal again, and within months, was well on her way. She skipped some classes, but instructed her sister-in-law, Martina, to get her homework from university professors. She made the dean's list.

By the time her 21st birthday came around, in March 2007, Katy had slogged through weeks of pain, doctors' appointments, hospital stays and trips to the operating room. She was down to 110 pounds from her typical 135 pounds. Her spirit not fully deflated, she kept her plans to go out to dinner and a night of bar-hopping to celebrate with a group of family and friends.

Kristy told her she needed a new outfit, and Katy agreed. Her old clothes were too big. She bought a pair of jeans and a pink tank top. She rounded out the outfit with a white, baby-doll style top. It was fashionable, yet Katy wore it not to be trendy, but to conceal a plastic bag hanging on her side.

The one-quart bag drained bile from her sick liver. She had carried it for several weeks. It was bulky, annoying and, as her mother put it, "just disgusting." As much as she tried to keep it empty, the bag seemed to fill up just as quickly as Katy got rid of its contents.

Katy's transplant coordinator had instructed her to measure the bile, reading the lines on the clear bag. Katy did so several times a day, dutifully writing the measurements in a spiral bound notebook. She squeezed the bag with her bare hands and emptied the bile into the toilet. She squirmed as the bile swirled in the commode. It was soupy and the color of fresh-cut grass.

"I want to get rid of this gross bag," she told Kristy as they prepared for the birthday night out.

The group's first stop was Bruno's, an Italian restaurant on Philadelphia Street, the main thoroughfare in downtown Indiana. The family sat in a wine cellar in the basement, the only room big enough for the large group. Katy picked at a piece of baked lasagna, her favorite dish.

"I'm not too hungry," she whispered to her mother, who sat across from her. "I'm so tired."

At Culpepper's, a bar adorned with portraits of Indiana native son Jimmy Stewart, Katy posed for photos with three of her brothers and other friends and family: Bryan, Josh, Jason, brother-in-law Scott, a family friend and previous crush named Brook, and Brad, who Katy had dated. The guys drank beers; Katy sipped on a cup of juice. One of her doctors had given her clearance to have one alcoholic drink and only one. She'd have it later.

The night picked up at Cozumel, a Mexican restaurant filled with the loud sounds of salsa music. The guys drank more, but the girls headed to the dance floor. Katy showed off some of her salsa moves. On the dance floor, Shelly held Katy's right hand with her left, placing her right hand around Katy's waist. Katy giggled as she put her left hand on Shelly's shoulder. Quick, quick, slow. Quick, quick, slow.

Katy's skin almost blended with the yellow walls in the background that displayed pictures of Mexico. But it was Katy's Liverpalooza, and damn it if she wasn't going to let loose and have fun. She wanted to show her illness that it could kiss her ass.

"I'm ready for my drink," she announced at Coney's, a popular bar in a building that once housed Indiana's first dry goods store.

Her mom and sisters had badgered her with suggestions on what to pick as her one drink, the one allowed by Dr. Kusum Tom, the surgeon following her treatment at the time. How about a Cosmopolitan, or a Long Island iced tea? A Zombie? No, a Flaming Dr. Pepper! Katy settled on a drink she'd had before, an apple martini.

She approached the bar with the determination of someone who's been there before. She sat on a stool next to Brad, flashing a smile as Martina snapped pictures. In less than a minute, the drink was gone. She downed it.

"Katy, it's not a shot!" Shelly warned. "You're supposed to sip it."

It was the moment she'd been waiting for months. For a brief moment, Katy forgot about the gross bag of bile, the itchy skin, the bloated belly, the yellow eyes. It was her moment, her birthday, her entrance into adulthood, into life as a woman eager to study, to marry and to live long.

She felt the bar spinning. Katy was tired. She'd danced, talked and drank, but Liverpalooza was catching up with her. She stepped away from the bar weak, her legs barely able to keep her upright. She felt a strong arm embrace her, hold her. Was it Brad? She smiled. It was Scott, Shelly's husband.

"I want to go home," she said.

"I'll walk you," Scott said.

The Irish music blared at Coney's as they left the bar and walked into the chilly night. It was a few minutes after midnight. Scott placed his right arm around Katy. His wife and sisters followed a few steps behind. Scott had watched Katy grow before his eyes like one of his own daughters. He felt overly protective, but knew there was nothing he could do about her illness. Happy birthday, my sweet Katy, he thought to himself.

He watched her in silence as he drove her home. Her eyes were closed. She was dreaming.

8

Complications

When Dr. Thomas Starzl encountered a complication in one of his patients, he solved the problem using a principle he learned from a scientific paper.

He believed a liver transplant could fail because of a technical mistake, a management problem or simply because the patient's underlying illness reared its ugly head.

It was a simple principle that seemed to make sense. Technical problems happen during the actual operation – opening up the abdomen, cutting out the sick liver and sewing in the new one.

The problem could happen right away, or set into motion a series of events that resulted in the problem days, weeks, months or even years later.

Management troubles emerge after the operation, such as when the right medication is not given at the right time, or waiting too long to fix a problem such as a biliary stricture.

And in some cases, Starzl believed, a liver illness roars back with a vengeance and obliterates any good that came out of the surgery. Nothing can be done about that.

In Katy's case, a peculiar combination of factors colluded to reduce her chances to get better.

Starzl figured out the problem early on. By the time Katy came along, he'd spent fifty years as the architect of the surgery she'd undergone. He knew liver surgery the way a car mechanic knows an engine tune-up.

Starzl checked on Katy every day, in the early morning and just before heading home. He drove his P.T. Cruiser to the top floor of the garage at UPMC Montefiore and stopped to get coffee in the lobby. He sat at the nurses' station, a grim look on his face, and examined any additions on Katy's medical record. Starzl was methodical in his examination. He took his time, often reading the same sentence more than once, as if trying to take a mental snapshot of the charts. He pored over cholangiograms, blood tests and biopsies and remembered key details, such as the measurement of albumin in her blood or if her blood was able to clot.

Instinctively, Starzl recognized Katy's bile duct had narrowed. To know for sure, he would have to see the liver with his naked eye and hold it in his own hands. Even without doing that, one thing was indisputable: the possibility of biliary strictures shouldn't be ignored.

The team assembled by Marcos and Starzl to work on the protocol held weekly meetings in a pathology conference room on the 7th floor of UPMC Montefiore. Nearly a dozen transplant experts pored over the records of the ten patients enrolled in the protocol. Sometimes it would take two hours for the surgeons and transplant coordinators to go over charts and test results. They talked about everything: whether an incision was healing well, whether a patient was sleeping through the night, or if their lab work was within acceptable ranges. Starzl never missed a meeting and decided this would be the perfect time to bring up his concerns to the group. He was blunt and straight forward and backed up everything he said with records and tests.

Marcos fumed at the implication that Katy's problems were caused by his management of the case, not an immunological problem. Starzl may have been a medical luminary, but he was not about to question Marcos' knowledge. Marcos had done more live-donor liver transplants than anyone in the world, and he wasn't about to be stepped on by anyone, not even Starzl.

"You don't understand live donor transplants," he barked at Starzl.

Starzl spent long hours at Montefiore, where nurses, residents and surgeons did not have to be reminded of his stature. What Starzl wanted, Starzl received. If something unusual went on, he almost always heard about it – all the more if it had something to do with one of the patients on the protocol.

It didn't take long for Starzl to uncover that other patients in the protocol were having trouble. The second patient, who followed Katy in February 2006, immediately experienced arterial complications. Another liver recipient, in September 2006, had to undergo surgery within a month of the transplant after experiencing a bile leak and biloma, an encapsulated collection of bile within the abdomen. Half of the ten patients in the protocol were experiencing complications of some sort or another. Starzl grew suspicious. Something was wrong and something had to be done.

It was late autumn 2006, when Katy was nearing the one-year anniversary of her transplant. Marcos kept busy with live-donor transplants; the thirty-six surgeries that year in Pittsburgh would be the most ever performed there in a one-year period.

Marcos had one other important project to complete: editing a 400-page reference book called "Living Donor Transplantation." The book, also edited by Drs. Henkie P. Tan and Ron Shapiro of the University of Pittsburgh, was meant to be an comprehensive guide to cellular and solid organ transplants.

One key chapter in the book, which would go on to be published in April 2007, reported a study of a subset of forty-seven patients in Pittsburgh who were on a specialized drug regimen. The study found biliary complications in 30 percent of recipients.

Tan asked Starzl to review the chapter, and as was practice in the preparation of scientific manuscripts, Starzl would be listed as an author for his collaboration.

Starzl jumped at the chance. It may have been pure coincidence, but getting his hands on the draft meant he could scrutinize details he was curious to know – the post-surgical outcomes of other live-donor liver transplant recipients in Pittsburgh.

"Terry, tell Henkie to send down the data," Starzl instructed his assistant, who within minutes fired off an email to Henkie Tan. Tan, who performed mostly kidney transplants, had been eager to position himself as a live-donor surgeon. He immediately complied with Starzl's request.

Starzl read the manuscript with the eye of a detective. He couldn't believe what he read, troubled by a nagging thought: How could the percentage of complications be so low at thirty percent, when he'd seen a higher percentage in the ongoing protocol?

Could it be Marcos? Starzl wondered. Never one to be outsmarted, Starzl and his research colleagues quickly sought to verify the data provided by Tan.

By December 2006, Starzl enlisted several university experts and examined details of every surgery performed by Marcos in Pittsburgh since his arrival in 2004.

The findings startled him: 65 percent of the 121 patients who'd undergone live donor liver transplants in Pittsburgh experienced a significant complication.

Starzl was furious. The findings were different from what anybody expected. He blamed Marcos.

"His personal behavior includes lying about complications," he would say later about Marcos in an interview with myself and another reporter for the *Pittsburgh Tribune-Review*.

Starzl's reaction was swift and pointed. He ordered Tan to take his name off the manuscript. He was not confrontational but, rather, practical: He didn't want his name on a chapter with potentially misleading information. That wasn't his style. Even more, he worried about the damage it could do to his reputation and his legacy.

Yet Starzl wasn't about to just let it end that way. Ever the mastermind, he agreed to write an introduction for the book, titled "Live Donor Transplantation: Then and Now." In it, Starzl and Marcos, as co-authors, explain the shift toward living donor transplantation as a way to address a shortage of dead donors.

Toward the end of the six-page introductory chapter, Starzl put the spotlight on Katy, although he didn't mention her by name. He declared the first five patients undergoing Katy's protocol had been successful, but wrote "the follow-ups are still too short to know whether this precise protocol is a definitive end to the search for the Holy Grail of organ tolerance or is only another step toward this objective."

Keeping his name on the book was a brilliant idea that would move the book forward – even with information he didn't believe to be true. It would be published, nonetheless, exposing Marcos and his data.

Marcos' book would show a low rate of complications when Starzl believed the reality was much different.

Even as Starzl appeared to support Marcos' book, he worked behind the scenes to notify university administrators of what was happening. He fired off letters to an internal university committee charged with overseeing quality assurance. Starzl just didn't want to report the problem – he wanted someone to fix it.

In disclosing the problem, Starzl cast a wide net: In a letter dated Dec. 12, 2006, he reported the problem to Jeffrey Romoff, the UPMC president. He wrote detailed descriptions of Katy's case and the rest of the protocol to Dr. Billiar, the chairman of surgery.

He told Billiar that as far back as August 2006, he'd urged Marcos to perform an ERCP, a procedure to inspect the bile ducts, but Marcos had declined. In November, a cholangiogram showed the telltale biliary obstruction. The "bile ducts were filled with insipissated bile that could not be removed," Starzl told the administrators.

Starzl wanted that reality to be public. He'd soon come up with a formidable plan to contradict the Marcos data: his own scientific paper revealing the true rate of complications. His papers always landed on the most prestigious medical journals. He'd find a way to tell the world.

9

Living pin cushion

The Millers' home smelled like ham, potatoes and broccoli casserole. It was Easter Sunday, and Kathy and Roger were hosting the family's traditional holiday gathering.

Kathy Miller woke up early that morning and headed straight to the kitchen. She'd made several jars of pickled eggs that she pulled from the refrigerator. The bright pink eggs were pickled in beet juice, the way her eight children liked them.

She poured the eggs from a tall glass jar and began slicing them on a cutting board. They were pickled all the way through the yolk, and she could see traces of pink around it. She put a slice in her mouth and grabbed another piece to take to Katy. Perfect, she thought to herself.

Katy was sleeping a few feet away in the living room. She'd drifted off early, groggy and with an empty stomach. A bowl of cold chicken broth sat on a tray table beside her. Kathy had pushed her to eat, but Katy refused. Her mother covered her yellow skin with a warm blanket.

"Try this, you'll like it," Kathy said, offering a small piece of egg. She wanted her to eat something, anything. For days, Katy had struggled to keep down any food. Broth and water was all she could stomach. Anything else, and her body revolted.

Politely, as always, Katy turned down the egg. She stayed on the couch as her family began to trickle in for the day. Nephews and nieces surrounded her, high on candy and ready to compete in the family's annual egg hunt.

It was a mild day for April, and Katy's brothers wore shorts and T-shirts. Every Easter they played hoops while the women cooked and set up the table. Katy moved from the couch only once, coaxed by her brother Jason to join the family at the dinner table.

She stared at her plate and barely touched the small slice of ham and spoonful of broccoli casserole her mother had served. She rubbed her swollen midsection the way a pregnant woman caresses her belly, as if she'd never noticed it before. She stood up as everyone stared and tried to pretend they weren't looking. But they were. They stole quick glances at the shrunken, tired, yellow person beside them. They pretended not to stare, but the picture before them was cruel, painful.

The liver Shelly had given Katy was supposed to make her better, not worse. Now here she was, shriveled, gaunt and tired. She was unable to eat, with a plastic bag of green bile on her belly and popping four Motrin pills three times a day, trying in vain to control the pain.

Katy returned to the couch and closed her eyes. She'd skipped Easter dinner, the egg hunt, and the basketball game in the sun. The

Millers carried on, eating, laughing, swearing. They checked on Katy periodically. Every once in a while, one of her brothers or sisters peeked in, nodding slightly, fixing her blanket, asking if there was anything she wanted to eat.

"You should stay here tonight," Kathy told Jason. Mother's intuition.

"Sure, Mom," he said.

By the time the family left, Jason found a spot on a couch next to Katy. The house was dark and the smell of baked ham lingered. Jason fell asleep, tired from a full day of eating and horsing around with his brothers. Just before 2 a.m. a distant thump awakened him. The noise came from the bathroom down the hall. Alarmed, Jason sat up and listened. He looked at the couch next to him. Katy was gone.

He stood up, walked to the bathroom, its door slightly open. He heard coughing.

"Hello?" Katy?" he said.

No answer.

"Katy? Is that you?"

He opened the door and found Katy slumped on the floor, her clothes covered in green bile and blood. His eyes traveled to the toilet. It looked as if someone had dumped in it a bucket of blood. Before reaching over for his sister, Jason yelled for his mom. Kathy didn't answer. He ran out of the bathroom and again called for his mother.

"Mom! She's vomiting blood!" he screamed, a rush of adrenaline coursing through his body. "Mom! Dad! Hurry!"

Jason Miller was scared. He'd watched his sister get sick over the past year, but she looked different this time. He propped Katy up on the floor; she felt lifeless. He patted her on the back, not knowing what else to do. *Are you OK? Are you OK?*

Kathy, half asleep and confused, called 911.

Katy arrived at Indiana Regional Medical Center at 2:20 a.m. Emergency doctors immediately transferred her by ambulance to UPMC Montefiore in Pittsburgh.

Dr. Linas Mockus was one of several doctors who examined Katy. His medical notes described Katy as slightly encephalopathic, a reference to dysfunction in her brain, but pleasant and able to carry a conversation. She didn't have a fever and complained of being thirsty. He noted that she had just experienced massive hemastosis, or vomiting of blood.

Dr. Mockus wrote: *I am seeing this critically ill patient status post living related liver transplantation on 11/1/2005 for the management of respiratory failure, renal failure, gastrointestinal bleeding, cholestasis, rejection and other complications after transplantation.*

Mockus intubated her and put her on a ventilator. He placed a central line in the left subclavian vein and consulted with other doctors, including liver transplant surgeons and hepatologists. They agreed Katy would undergo an upper gastrointestinal endoscopy to determine why she was vomiting blood and where it was coming from. During the procedure, Dr. Kapil Chopra inserted a scope through Katy's mouth, all the way down to the descending part of the small intestine, the portion in which the bile ducts empty.

There were four columns of grade 3 to grade 4 esophageal varices starting in the mid esophagus extending into the distal esophagus. At least two of the esophageal variceal columns had stigmata of recent bleeding in the form of hematocystic spots. There was a superficial ulceration overlying two of the esophageal varices. There was no evidence of any fresh or active bleeding during the procedure.

Esophageal varices – swollen veins in the lower part of the esophagus near the stomach – are common in people like Katy with serious liver disease. Because the blood flow to the liver has been impaired, the blood backs into surrounding blood vessels, making them swell and looking like varicose veins that some people have in their legs. Like hemorrhoids, esophageal varices can balloon to the point where they rupture. The varices found in the lining of Katy's esophagus, grade 3 and grade 4, were the largest. At grade 4, there is a severe threat of impending hemorrhage.

Katy's examination found two more columns of varices in the cardia, the part of the stomach attached to the esophagus. In the stomach, Chopra found evidence of portal hypertensive gastropathy, another sign that her liver was on the precipice of failure. The lining of Katy's stomach was covered with distended blood vessels, something caused by the increased pressure on her portal vein.

Chopra used a common procedure called band ligation to fix the varices. He wrapped three rubber bands around the three large columns of varices that ran up and down the esophagus. The procedure was successful and, in his medical notes, Chopra noted that the varices had been decompressed and there was no evidence of bleeding.

Katy's level of bilirubin was 22, more than ten times the normal 2. Her creatinine level was 5.1, a sky-high number that shows a person at the tipping point of renal failure. Her kidneys were shutting down fast, unable to remove waste from the blood and losing their filtering capacity. Every day, the kidneys process 200 quarts of blood to sift out about two quarts of waste products and extra water. Katy couldn't do this. They'd have to put her on a dialysis machine to take over for her failing kidneys.

Katy's mother had never seen her daughter this sick, and she went to great lengths to explain to me how Easter Day became a turning point for the entire family. Before the transplant, Katy battled nausea, diarrhea and stomach pain, but she had never been so weak and so miserable. Katy had retained so much fluid, her skin seeped fluid. Her sister Shelley watched in disbelief as she touched Katy's skin and could see droplets of water oozing out.

To see Katy so sick now, when she had never been sick before the transplant, unleashed a torrent of questions that always led to the same path: Did Katy really need the transplant to begin with?

Kathy, by then intimately familiar with the changes in her daughter's body, knew that was a moot point. Katy was sick *now,* and something had to be done. She spoke daily to Caponi, the registered nurse who was Katy's transplant coordinator. No one doubted Caponi's good intentions and her always candid assessments delivered with a throaty smoker's voice. She was intense and tender at the same time.

"I think she needs another liver," Kathy told Caponi.

Kathy knew her daughter was as close as she'd ever been to death, but neither Kathy, nor anyone else in the family, was ready to concede defeat. Her daughter was too sick to make a decision on her own and the family felt obligated to act on her behalf, even if Katy was twenty-one.

Caponi gave the Millers as much information as she could, but not enough to satisfy Kathy. In the hours after Katy had been admitted to Montefiore, she'd been poked and probed so many times that Kathy thought her daughter was a medical guinea pig.

"She was a living pin cushion," she would tell me later in one of our many conversations.

During a visit with a pastor from her hometown, Katy held hands with her mother and prayed.

"Don't worry about me," Katy told him.

Politely, Katy asked if he could add another person to his prayer list. It was Michelle Wine, a twenty-seven-year-old woman that Katy had met at the hospital. They bumped into each other while buying snacks at the hospital gift shop. Katy and Michelle struck up a conversation and discovered both were waiting for a liver transplant. Katy was waiting for her second liver, Michelle for her third.

Katy and Michelle became fast friends. On clinic days, they ate breakfast together in the hospital cafeteria. If they weren't hungry, they sipped on bottled water or hot tea while they talked. They listened to each other gripe about their doctors, the long wait for a transplant and the incessant itching. They found comfort knowing that both felt like bugs were constantly crawling on their skin.

If Katy was too sick, Michelle would beg her mother to take her to Katy's hospital room. When Katy was moved to an isolation room on the 12th floor, Michelle donned a mask and gown. The two friends held hands and prayed for each other. Katy often went to Michelle's room, wearing a surgical mask and pajamas.

"You're going to get your liver," Katy would tell Michelle over and over.

As she watched Katy turn more yellow, Kathy pressed doctors for answers. Her illness just came back, she remembers them saying. Kathy never knew much about PSC but no one could dispute that Katy's new liver was failing. How else could you explain her yellow skin, the bloated belly, the failing kidneys? *Why aren't they putting her on the waiting list for another liver?*

Kathy became increasingly distraught and grew suspicious of every decision doctors made. Even Starzl, who had developed a strong bond with Katy and Shelly, seemed more secretive. He had suddenly altered the timing of his visits to Katy's hospital room. Instead of showing up in the late morning or in the afternoon, he arrived early, before the daylight nursing shift took over.

Wearing a suit and tie, he'd walk into Katy's room and close the door behind him. He'd pull up a chair and sit by her bedside. He'd reach for her hand. She'd open her eyes and he smiled. *Is that Starzl?* She smiled, too, asking how he was.

He looked her in the eyes, yellow like a wilted daffodil, bothered that her new liver was failing. *She needs to get back on the list.*

Kathy and other relatives spoke to nurses, doctors and other workers in the ICU, and were very much aware a serious dispute had emerged between Starzl and Marcos. The conflict confused them, making the family all the more tense. *Who should we trust? Who's telling the truth?*

Kathy's level of distrust increased during a conversation with Dr.

Kusum Tom, one of the surgeons who operated on Katy. As Kathy remembers it, Dr. Tom gave her the impression that her daughter could have been relisted in the fall of 2006, when she became jaundiced and bile duct problems emerged.

I spoke to several people involved in Katy's case about the timing of her listing for a second transplant. They agreed there might have been resistance to putting her back on the list because it would have represented not only the failure of her first transplant, but also the failure of the protocol. Yet, they were clear that no one at UPMC would have done anything to harm Katy.

"Marcos would never intentionally harm anyone," Caponi said. "Marcos didn't have bad intentions. He did what he thought was best."

When I reviewed Katy's medical records, which Kathy requested from UPMC at a cost of more than $200 that I paid, some entries showed Katy had been relisted at the time of her Easter hospitalization in April 2007.

On account of her worsening jaundice and organ function, the patient is currently relisted for liver transplantation, Chopra wrote on the April 9 notes.

Kathy disputed the records. She told me that in a conversation with Caponi a few days after Katy's admission, she had to threaten Marcos to get Katy back on the list.

"Tell Marcos if she's not on the transplant list tomorrow morning, we're moving out and transferring Katy to another hospital," Kathy said she told Caponi, well aware there were other transplant programs in town, but unsure if she had the guts to carry through with her threat.

If the medical records were correct, and Katy had been relisted before Easter, why did Dr. Tom tell Kathy her daughter should have been relisted sooner? Could it have been that Dr. Tom was unaware of Katy's relisting? Or was the physician simply trying to empathize with the family?

"My memory is shot," Tom told me later. "All I know is that at the time nobody wanted to admit failure."

On the morning after Kathy spoke with Caponi, Marcos showed up in Katy's hospital room. He sat next to Kathy, but she didn't say a word. She just glared at him.

"I've decided to put you back on the waiting list," he announced.

"OK," Katy mumbled, not looking at him, not looking at anything.

In the throes of a protocol that once promised to revolutionize transplantation, Marcos now faced a new test. With Katy's case on the brink of disaster, he was jockeying to save the protocol with nine other patients who had also been transplanted.

Marcos looked at Katy's mother, searching for a nod or a word of acceptance. She offered nothing but dagger eyes. The blame for Katy's downward spiral needed to fall somewhere. Marcos became the target of the family's hatred. Katy, her mind clouded by painkillers, fired verbal bombs that drew laughs from her brothers.

"What are you doing here?" Katy had screamed the minute Marcos walked into her hospital room. "You are such a douche bag!"

Katy slurred her words, but they came out like a speeding fist, like a sucker punch. Her brothers lost it when they heard her, a mixture of approval and solidarity. *Douche bag!* There was nothing they could do but laugh, blaming it on the drugs, but knowing full well that their sister meant every bit of it.

Katy was no longer the sweet, innocent girl Marcos paraded as a career trophy. Her personality had changed. She had an attitude and wasn't afraid to speak her mind. But she was no longer healthy and vibrant. She was a yellow, withering flower. *Douche bag.* That's all he deserved.

"I like your jeans," she told Marcos one weekend as he walked into the room, casually dressed. "But don't you think they're too tight?"

A week after she was listed for a second liver, a doctor walked into the ICU. He hurried into Katy's room and found her in the bathroom.

"Get her off there," the man said. "We have a new liver."

He was looking at a picture of the liver on a cell phone. *A liver. A new liver.* The words were so unexpected that Kathy didn't know what to make of them. She knew her daughter was dying and needed a new liver. Yet what she learned about the organ donor gave her pause. This time, Katy's new liver wouldn't come from Shelly. The liver came from a stranger they knew little about.

All the Miller family knew was that the liver came from a 300-pound woman. Katy, who at her heaviest weighed no more than 135 pounds, was probably down to a hundred pounds. A tiny body for what was likely a much bigger organ.

Marcos had talked to me about the difficulties of using large organs on smaller patients during an interview in which we spoke about the shortage of organs for transplantation. The obesity epidemic in the United States has caused the increase of an illness known as nonalcoholic steatohepatitis. He told me it was a common and often silent condition that can lead to liver failure. People who suffer from it have excessive fat in the liver, along with inflammation and damage. More people had livers that are often twice as large as those of average size.

"So what do you do with an organ?" Marcos asked me. "Essentially first you won't be able to fit it into someone that's small, you just can't close the abdomen. It becomes a problem."

Such a statement wouldn't have mattered to Katy. At this stage of the game, she wanted to live.

"Are you sure of this, Katy? I don't know about this," Kathy said, a strange sensation washing through her.

"Yes, I want it," Katy said.

Nurses whisked Katy away to the surgical preparation area in a matter of minutes. Kathy immediately called Shelly, who was in a waiting room down the hall. Kathy wondered why no one had asked her if she agreed to the surgery. Then it hit her. They didn't need her permission. Katy was an adult, old enough to decide her own fate.

"I don't care, Mom. It's a liver. I want it," Katy said one last time.

□ □ □ □ □ □ □

Katy's second transplant presented a unique opportunity for Starzl.

He had known all along what was wrong with Katy's liver: Biliary strictures were suffocating her bile ducts and as a result, destroying the liver she had received from her sister seventeen months before.

Starzl's insight came from ultrasounds and cholangiograms, all of which he had reviewed and all of which provided detailed images of Katy's liver. He also knew that Katy's immunosuppressive regime had been altered with no significant effect. She'd been given prednisone and other drugs, but they were not able to stop her liver's rapid deterioration.

There was no question in his mind as to what was causing such a precipitous downfall, but Thomas Starzl was a stubborn man. The ultimate confirmation could be obtained only one way – if he could examine Katy's liver with his own hands, once surgeons pulled it out of her body during the second transplant.

Leave it to Starzl to come up with a way to do just that.

Once removed in the OR, the liver would be placed on a metal tray to be delivered to a pathology laboratory. A technician would inspect it, take pictures, write a detailed description and finally slice it. In inch-thick sections, he would chop up the liver that Shelly had given to her sister. The technician would arrange the pieces of the liver on slides to be inspected under a microscope by a pathologist.

Starzl was determined to see Katy's liver before it was sliced. He wanted to hold it, touch it and inspect the bile ducts with his own eyes – the eagle eyes that he used for years to cut and sew livers and kidneys in dogs and in humans. For a man like Starzl, recognized and respected by everyone at Montefiore, getting his hands on this liver wasn't a difficult task.

As soon as Starzl got word that Katy was headed to the operating room to get a new liver, he called the technician and informed him he'd be coming in. He arrived within thirty minutes and put on a pair of surgical gloves. He'd worn them thousands of times before when he was transplant king and saving lives.

Starzl lifted Katy's liver and examined it. It weighed three pounds, thirteen ounces, just about average. He didn't use a microscope or a magnifying glass; he touched the bile ducts and felt the gravel clogged in their nooks and crannies.

"Look at that," he pointed again and again. "Look at that."

Starzl had what he needed – the truth, his truth, the final validation of what led to the failure of Katy's promising protocol. Starzl may have been in his eighties, but in many ways, this was a war unlike anything he'd experienced in his career.

Marcos had argued that Katy had encountered an immunological setback, one caused by the drugs she was taking, but Starzl now believed he had evidence to dispute that. Starzl believed the obstruction in Katy's biliary tract was a management issue that could have been fixed.

Katy's official pathology report, signed by Dr. Anthony J. Demetris, director of transplantation pathology at UPMC Montefiore, stated: *"The primary cause of the liver allograft failure is extra- and intra-hepatic biliary tract ulcerations and strictures (radiographic) with small bile duct loss and extensive portal vein branch obliteration, which correlates clinically with the hyperbilirubinemia and portal hypertension/ascites."*

Katy's liver had been labeled with her initials, KM, and the words "allograft liver." It was twenty-four centimeters long, eighteen centimeters wide and eight centimeters deep.

Demetris' report provided succinct, but revealing summary of Katy's case, starting with the transplant on the day after Halloween 2005. Katy's immunosuppression had been minimized four months after the surgery. Two months later, her blood work began to show higher than normal levels of liver enzymes. Liver biopsies during that time showed evidence of a mild rejection reaction and over a period of several months, "increasingly severe changes of biliary tract obstruction/structuring." The biliary strictures eventually were documented using an X-ray examination and portal hypertension developed, the report said.

Demetris wrote that the underlying cause of the biliary tract injury, or strictures, could not be determined with absolute certainty by just examining the liver under the microscope. However, he offered more than one contributing factor: "an anastomotic stricture related to suboptimal healing of the mucosa at that site, antibody and/or cell mediated rejection, and recurrence of the original disease."

After his initial slide review, Demetris held extensive discussions with Starzl about the biliary tract stricture, he wrote. It had been Starzl's opinion, Demetris wrote, that "suboptimal vascularization of the distal biliary tree and anastomotic stricturing was the major underlying cause of the biliary strictures and all other changes were secondary to that process." Starzl's conclusion honed in on the Achilles' Heel of a liver transplant – that surgeons, no matter how skilled, are unable to predict the level of blood supply that can be restored throughout the new organ.

Demetris, however, could not rule out other factors that may have contributed to the liver's failure. He explained that PSC developed in such a way that he could not definitely exclude the possibility that it may have contributed to the biliary injury. He supported this by noting that there was biochemical evidence of strictures six months after the transplant as well as injury and ulceration of the bile ducts.

Starzl didn't believe this. Convinced of his conclusion, he took his findings to Dr. Richard Simmons, UPMC Presbyterian's chief of quality assurance and Billiar, the chief of surgery at the University of Pittsburgh. Both agreed the matter should be presented at a clinical pathological conference, where other surgeons and pathologists could review and discuss its details.

Marcos did not attend the meeting. Instead, he sent Paulo Fontes, the surgeon who had first met with Katy about a potential transplant more than a year before. Despite Starzl's standing as the father of transplantation and his title of Distinguished Service Professor of Surgery, Fontes questioned his presentation.

Starzl screamed at Fontes: "This is a biliary stricture that wasn't treated!"

In Starzl's view, waiting to treat the problem had ruined Katy's transplanted liver. I spoke to several people who suggested that by the time Marcos acted to correct the biliary stricture, it was too late. Strictures are often unavoidable. But you have to recognize them and fix them early on.

It is impossible to know if Marcos purposely stalled. Was he concerned about Katy's survival, and not so much about her complications? UNOS, after all, tracks patient survival, not surgical complications. Was Marcos simply intent on showing above-average survival, regardless of how well the patient was doing? I repeatedly reached out to him, trying to get an answer. Marcos never called me back.

UPMC leaders, already aware of Starzl's disapproval of Marcos' transplant outcomes, stood by Marcos' clinical judgment and rebuffed Starzl for questioning his authority. Within twelve hours of the meetings, administrators cut off Starzl's access to all patient medical records.

□ ❏ □ ❏ □ ❏ □

The second transplant improved Katy's bilirubin levels. They had been measured as high as 30 milligrams per deciliter, when normal levels typically range from 0.3 to 1.9.

But by its very nature, retransplantation comes with a higher risk of infection and a higher risk of technical complications. While Katy's blood pressure stabilized and her liver panels showed a slight improvement, she spent the days after the transplant sleeping and barely able to move from her hospital bed. She lost interest in watching television or reading books.

When I spoke to Shelly about the second transplant and its aftermath, she spoke about a version of Katy that hardly resembled the Katy I had met, or the ebullient college student whose heart had captivated her family and her friends.

"She loved every one of us, but she was tired and fed up," Shelly told me. "She had lost her will. She was frustrated."

It bothered Katy that she had no say in anything her doctors and nurses did to her. If they needed to test her blood, they pricked her and probed her until they could get what they wanted. *A living pin cushion.* Katy just wanted them to ask if it was OK to touch her, jab her with needles and fill her with blood transfusions. She didn't want them to assume she had given her consent to having strange hands prod and turn her like a side of beef.

"I'm done," Katy had told her sister. "If I get this second transplant, and it doesn't work, that's it. This will be my last."

Shelly, whose own belly was marked by a long incision where doctors took part of her liver, became a constant presence at the hospital. She brought books for her sister and kept her up-to-date on family stories. Scott, her husband, stood at the end of the hospital bed and massaged Katy's legs.

When more relatives showed up, they ordered take-out from one of the nearby restaurants in Oakland. They'd hand Katy a menu, always mindful to include her. She'd take a long time studying every single description and struggled to make a selection. When her food finally came, she wouldn't eat it.

Kathy often spent the night at the hospital, struggling to fall asleep on a chair, an ever-vigilant mother looking after her child. Katy never asked anyone to stay with her. *Would you like someone to stay?* her mother would ask. *Yes*, Katy said.

"She was as sick as any person could be without dying," Kathy would tell me later.

On the first weekend of May 2007, Kathy stayed home with the flu, too sick to drive to the hospital. She worried she would pass on her germs to Katy, whose immune system was already depleted. The rest of the family took over, sitting in the hospital room watching Katy, waiting for any sign of a turnaround.

"My legs are hairy," Katy told Shelly. It was a warm, sunny day, the type of day that typically boosted Katy's spirits.

"I'll shave them for you," Shelly said.

Shelly didn't have a razor and left the room in search of one. She walked to the nurses' station, where a kind nurse offered a razor wrapped in a clear bag. Shelly placed a plastic chair under the shower in the bathroom that was part of Katy's hospital room. She wheeled in Katy and pushed up her pajama gown, careful not to get it wet. She leaned Katy's back on the chair and gently washed her long, black hair, which was crusty and matted to her head. One by one, Shelly lifted Katy's legs, slathered them with shaving cream and shaved them. It feels good, Katy told her.

"Let's go outside," Shelly suggested. "It's bright and sunny. It will make you feel better."

It sounded like a great idea. In the weeks since the second transplant, Katy had been confined to her room, tempted by the warmer days of late spring. On a day like this, she would have been studying for finals at college, probably in her bedroom at her parents' house in Creekside, alone but safe and alive. *A living pin cushion*, that's what she was now.

Shelly dried Katy's hair and brushed it. By the time she was done, Jason had popped in and talked about his night at the bar with Scott. Often times, Jason would stay at a hotel near the hospital so he could be near his sister. He was happy to see Katy so willing to get some sunlight.

"I can't wait to get out of here," she said, still in her pajamas, still yellow. "I hate this place."

Jason pushed Katy's wheelchair out of her room, and Shelly and Bryan walked behind them. They took the elevator to the lobby and walked to the hospital's main entrance. The sliding glass door opened and Katy felt the sun on her face for the first time in weeks. Jason parked the wheelchair by the flag pole. The sky was a bright sapphire blue, a welcome change from the fluorescent hospital lights.

Katy found herself with a full view of the cloudless sky. The disgust that overwhelmed Katy throughout her hospital stay suddenly lifted. She felt a tickle on her throat and spit on the cement.

She was happy. She wanted to go home.

10

"No, not my baby!"

On Monday, May 7, 2007, exactly seventeen days after her second liver transplant, Katy sat on her hospital bed, pulled the blanket off her legs and asked her mother for help to go to the bathroom. She seemed disoriented and mumbled her words.

Prograf, she said, referring to the anti-rejection medicine she had been taking the last year and a half.

"Why don't we go to Hoss's for lunch?" Katy said to her mother, not making much sense.

Kathy stared at her daughter – the yellow skin, the bloated belly, the messy mane of black hair. For the last month, Katy had been trapped in a hospital, and for the last month, every breath, every scan and every blood draw had been closely monitored by Montefiore's highly skilled transplant surgeons.

"I'm hoping she'll go home by Friday," Kathy had told her husband a few minutes before.

By the time she made it back to her bed from the bathroom, Katy was hanging on to her mother's shoulder. She was weak and couldn't breathe. She needed help. A critical care doctor, Ali Al-Khafaji, arrived in the room within minutes and found her sitting in bed. He measured Katy's respiratory rate at thirty to thirty-five breaths per minute, higher than the normal twelve to twenty breaths. He immediately transferred her to the transplant intensive care unit on the fifth floor. They put her in Bed Number 23.

Al-Khafaji lifted Katy's hospital gown and examined her distended belly. It was tense to touch, filled with excess fluid, much as it had been over the past several days, according to his progress notes. He needed to relieve the pressure. He'd do it the same way doctors have done it for years – using a pigtail catheter with a curved tip.

Guiding himself with an ultrasound, he inserted a fourteen-gauge needle into Katy's abdomen and threaded a small wire through it. He took out the needle, and put the catheter with the tightly curled end over the wire. Slowly, he drained from her belly a turbid, extremely yellow fluid. Doing this, he hoped, would improve Katy's breathing.

Before he left the room, Al-Khafaji instructed another doctor to disconnect her PICC line, afraid the catheter might be infected, even though there were no traces of blood in the fluid. Kathy waited outside. She tried to call Shelly. She could hear alarms going off in Katy's room.

"You better get here fast," she told Shelly, who was taking a walk with friends and was about forty-five minutes away from the hospital.

Katy's breathing worsened. Al-Khafaji returned, this time doing a STAT echocardiogram to get a quick look at her heart. What he saw wasn't good: there was a significant amount of fluid building up around her heart. And there was a chance it could be blood. Whatever it was, it was compressing the heart, keeping it from pumping enough blood to the lungs and the rest of the body.

Within seconds, doctors put a tube down her windpipe, hooked her to a mechanical ventilator and scrambled to drain the fluid building around her heart. Katy, however, was unresponsive. She didn't have a pulse. Someone performed CPR. An ultrasound showed a distended, engorged right internal jugular vein – tell-tale evidence that fluid was squashing her heart. A fellow stuck a needle into her chest, straight into the sac that holds the heart and the roots of the great vessels. He drew large amounts of dark, bloody fluid: first about two tablespoons, then nearly a cup. By the time he was done, he had collected nearly ten times the amount of fluid that normally surrounds the heart muscle.

Katy regained her pulse, only to lose it again. They were losing her. They stuffed her with drugs in a desperate attempt to increase her heart rate: 10 ampules of epinephrine, 4 grams of calcium chloride, 10 ampules of sodium bicarbonate, 40 units of vasopressin. When her hemoglobin collapsed, they pumped her with 10 liters of blood. The CPR continued.

Down the hall in a waiting room, Kathy had no idea what was happening. She struck up a conversation with the wife of a man who'd also had a liver transplant. The woman was outgoing and cheerful and told Kathy not to worry. Her husband had fluid drained from his abdomen four or five times before and had been fine. They sat side-by-side, and her friendliness comforted Kathy. Another hour went by and Kathy peeked down the long hallway. She noticed commotion outside Room 23.

A resident stopped her from walking further, nearly pushing her back into a narrow room near the nurses' station. She knew the room all too well; others had told her it was the room where people got bad news.

Al-Khafaji suddenly appeared out of nowhere. He sat next to her, grabbing her hand.

"We tried as hard as we could," he said.

It was 3:04 p.m. Katy was dead.

Kathy doesn't remember what happened afterward. At some point, she went outside for air and threw up in the hospital driveway.

Al-Khafaji's notes were winding and clinical. "I explained to her that this resuscitation is futile and that we are not sure that continuing to do CPR is going to help, especially at the end even with CPR and with maximum amounts of vasopressors and inotropes, the patient did not regain her spontaneous circulation."

In his notes, filed that night around 8 p.m., Al-Khafaji wrote: "It was quite unclear what exactly the problem was and why this patient deteriorated so quickly. She clearly has multiple medical problems and clearly had multiple causes that could have led to her demise; however, we were quite distressed by the fact that these events happened quite quickly."

News of Katy's death spread quickly throughout the transplant center. Nurses, aides and transplant coordinators openly cried, hugging each other. Shelly, who had arrived minutes before, called her father, who was driving his pickup truck near Creekside. Before she said anything about Katy, Shelly asked him to pull over.

"No! Not my baby!" Roger Miller sobbed on the phone. He

became so distraught that Shelly had to ask a friend to pick him up and drive him to the hospital. She called her four brothers and two other sisters.

In the confusing moments that followed, a nurse asked the family if they wanted to go see Katy's body. Shelly and Kristy briefly hesitated, looked at each other, and walked into Room 23. Katy was covered with a blanket up to her chest. Her eyes were closed and her hands rested on her stomach. Her face was discolored, her black hair matted to her head. Blood trickled from her nose and mouth, down to her cheeks, her neck.

"Can someone clean her up?" Shelly screamed at no one in particular. "Wipe that blood off her face!"

She nearly banged on the gurney, but Kristy stopped her. Both sisters cried as they watched a nurse wipe Katy's face with a wet towel. Small trickles of blood came out again. The nurse explained the blood was normal because of transfusions Katy had received in a short time – more than double the average four liters of a typical case.

The sisters almost didn't notice when Starzl walked in, his wrinkled hands in his pockets, his head downward. He stood in the corner and looked around. He approached Kathy, tapped her on the arm and reached to embrace her. The father of transplantation, eighty years old and counting, cried.

As upset as he was, there was something he wanted to tell the Millers. We need to find out what happened, he told them. Starzl urged the Millers to authorize an autopsy, something Katy's father opposed. There were a lot of questions about her death, and Starzl wanted answers. For him, for them, for everyone.

"She's been through enough," Roger Miller told Starzl.

Two days later, on May 9, 2007, Starzl sent a letter to Dr. Richard Simmons, UPMC Presbyterian's chief of quality assurance. It read in part:

"For the following reason, I was ashamed of the UPMC liver program in which I once took such pride. The diagnosis and treatment of this young woman's complication had been actively prevented by the chief of transplant surgery until it was too late."

I called Marcos repeatedly to talk about Starzl's comments. On one occasion, he told me he'd talk to me. He later backed out.

□ □ □ □ □ □ □

I met Michelle Wine, Katy's friend, at the same sandwich shop where I had met Starzl a few weeks before. Michelle had just left the transplant clinic, and when I approached her, she was on her cell phone, arguing with a drugstore clerk over who'd pay for her anti-rejection medicine.

"You don't fill my prescription and I die, you understand?" she said with a quivering voice. "I don't have two hundred dollars to put out every month."

Michelle was small and skinny, with arms so bony and fragile I thought they might break if anyone touched them. She'd been born with an illness called cholestasis, which blocked the flow of bile to her liver.

"I feel like I've had so much taken away from me," she told me with a level of maturity that I had not expected.

The illness caused her to be so yellow that other children laughed and pointed at her at the swimming pool.

"Look at that monster!" she'd hear them say.

Her itching became so severe at times, she'd have to be taken to the hospital because no medicine would make it stop. When she met Katy, she was happy to meet someone who could empathize with her, who could understand her pain, who could listen to her.

By the time she was twenty-one, Michelle had received two transplants. That was when she started having problems again. She threw up constantly and picked up one infection after another. She became so sick she had to put her schooling on hold; she'd been going to a community college, trying to get a nursing degree.

She waited for 18 ½ months for her third liver. The surgery didn't solve her problems. Doctors blasted her with steroids to fight the almost immediate rejection. They put Benadryl straight into her veins to stop the itching. She cried herself to sleep many nights, wondering if she would ever receive another transplant. It finally came, her fourth one, in September 2008.

Yet, here she was, still alive, still able to tell her story, and unlike Katy, still able to worry about the future. At first, Michelle's mother hid from her the news about Katy's death. Michelle knew something was wrong, but her mother wouldn't tell her. Michelle was too sick, in desperate need of a new liver.

The new organ finally came. Within a few days Michelle felt strong enough to walk around the intensive care unit.

"I want to see Katy," she told her mother.

"OK, you can see Katy," her mother said, knowing full well Katy had died.

She changed the subject, but Michelle insisted she wanted to see Katy. Her mother finally confessed.

"Katy didn't make it," she said.

Michelle cried as she never had before, holding on to her belly because her incisions were still fresh and raw.

"She wouldn't want you to be upset," her mother said.

As she recalled the story, Michelle began to cry and wipe her tears. I pictured Katy and Michelle holding hands in the hospital room, leaning on each other, praying and wondering if they would ever get out of there.

"Oh my God, here I am, I'm alive, I made it through this," she told me. "Is this going to happen to me? Am I going to die?"

Michelle remained resentful and hurt because she never said goodbye to Katy. She taped a picture of Katy on a mirror in her bedroom. She often holds it, looking at it, and just bawls, she told me.
"Why did it have to be you?" she'd say to herself.

Just as quickly, however, she told me she has a purpose. She doesn't know what it is, but she vowed to find out. There must be a reason why she is alive and Katy is not.

Her fourth liver is giving her problems. Her portal vein – which carries blood into the liver from the stomach, intestines, spleen, gallbladder, and pancreas – once became clogged and doctors have talked about propping it open with a stent.

"I believe she's with me in spirit," Michelle told me about Katy. "I miss her every day."

As hard as Katy fought, Michelle said Katy was tired of taking medicine and hated everything about going to the hospital: the drive, the long hallways, the sterile rooms, the constant probing of her body.

We were just about to end our conversation when I looked up and noticed Starzl appear from out of nowhere with a lunch tray. He was placing it on a table not too far from ours when I told Michelle he was there. He had performed her first two transplants when she was barely a child. He had retired by the time she had her fourth transplant in September 2008.

Michelle stood up and approached Starzl. He recognized her instantly and the two embraced. Michelle seemed almost lost in his arms.

"I'm here because of you," she said, tears rolling down her cheeks.

They spoke briefly, and I tried not to listen, wondering how Starzl managed to remember every one of his patients, no matter their age or their hometown. When they were done talking, he said goodbye to both of us and told us he'd take his lunch tray to another table so that Michelle and I could finish our conversation.

I asked about her other doctors, and she spoke about them the way most people speak about their grade-school teachers, with admiration, gratitude and respect. She mentioned each by name, fast and assured, as if to tell me that she was well aware of what they did and how much value she placed on their care.

"I can't say anything bad about them," she said. "If these doctors wouldn't fight for me, I wouldn't be here."

"I think that when it's your time, it's your time," she told me. "For some reason, God called her."

□ ❑ □ ❑ □ ❑ □

On June 25, 2007, forty-five days after Katy died, I received an email from Kristy:

Hello Luis,

This is Kristy Miller, one of Katy Miller's sisters. You did an article on Katy a while back about her liver transplant and her disease PSC. Since then Katy has passed and I was wondering if there was any way to get a copy of the article.

Thank you,

Kristy Miller

Katy Miller was dead? The beautiful college student whose case Amadeo Marcos had trumpeted was *dead?* The important protocol he told me would guarantee quality of life for Katy had failed? *This will change transplantation. Quality of life. Quality of life is the goal.*

It took me several minutes to understand Kristy's email. I read it several times, slowly, line by line, word by word, looking for an opening, an error. Did I understand this right? *Since then Katy has passed.*

I replied as soon as my fingers let me. *Oh my goodness, I didn't know Katy had passed away. When did this happen? I am so sorry to hear that. She was such an inspiring young woman. Please tell your family how bad I feel and extend my sympathies. I will try to find a copy of the newspaper. I can also try to get you some prints of the photos we ran, because I thought they were really nice. Please send me the address where I can send them.*

It took her all day to reply, and I wondered if I had said something wrong in my note. Had I not been sympathetic enough? I reread the words I wrote. They seemed harmless enough. When she wrote, Kristy apologized for the delay. She was writing from Harrisburg, where she was working in an Army barracks, helping to gather supplies for soldiers who would soon be leaving for Iraq.

Yes, she passed on May 7th from complications after her second liver transplant. It was very sudden and very hard. Thank you for your sympathy. Katy was my best friend, hell she was everyone's best friend. Everything about that little girl was infectious from her smile to her looks on to her personality and heart. She was as beautiful inside as out, and I miss her so much every day. I got on the computer and Googled her name just to see what would come up. The article with that picture just reminded me of all that shit (excuse my language) that she had to go through and how she was promised she was in the best care. So, I would love to thank you for getting back to me. Sorry if I am rambling...

It wasn't until several months later that I started piecing together the Katy Miller puzzle. It had never occurred to me that her case had led to the derailment of the Marcos-Starzl protocol. The story crystallized when I worked on an investigation about liver transplants on people who don't need them. Unlike Katy's case, that series focused on people who received organs from deceased donors. But Katy's story had been mentioned by several surgeons as an example of the philosophical, and perhaps seismic, transformation taking place in Pittsburgh, where surgeons had once strictly focused on first giving new organs to the sickest patients and now did not.

We'd just begun working on the investigative piece when it occurred to me that I should talk to Katy's mother. I had met her in 2006, but didn't have her phone number. I emailed Kristy, and she responded within a few hours. *She would love to talk you about the subject.*

11

80 years worth of living

The pink lipstick looked too gaudy on Katy's lips. Her body had been placed in a casket, and Kristy and Carol, her sister-in-law, concluded the bright pink shade wasn't elegant enough for Katy.

The basement at the Moore & Moore funeral home in Indiana seemed dark and damp. The caretaker had escorted Kristy and Carol downstairs, hoping they would approve of the way he had prepared Katy's body.

Katy's body was puffy, her black hair unwilling to lay the right way. She was dressed in an outfit selected by her sisters: a black blouse and silk pants. As they approached Katy, lifeless and stiff, Kristy and Carol clung to each other.

They sobbed, shaking as they tried to compose themselves. All that was left of Katy was in a box, and they struggled to understand how unfair it seemed. The more they stared at her, the more questions they had. Katy was supposed to be a promising college student, not a corpse in the basement of a funeral home.

Part of Kristy felt indignant standing before her dead sister, but she was overcome by a feeling of sadness and futility. Almost instinctively, she wiped off the pink lipstick with a tissue. Tears were rolling down her cheeks, but Kristy was laughing inside because Katy would have never worn a bright pink lipstick like that. Not when she was alive, and most certainly not when she was dead.

Using a pair of scissors they found on a nearby table, Kristy cut several lockets of Katy's hair. Carol wrapped them in paper and stuffed them in her purse. Kristy reached to Katy's hands, studying her sister's fingernails. Now, *that* needs some color, she said to Carol. She produced a bottle of nail polish and spent the next several minutes painting Katy's fingernails.

They tried to brush Katy's hair but it wouldn't cooperate. She doesn't look like Katy, Kristy kept thinking, internalizing a mix of anger and denial. She called her mother, who had been waiting upstairs. They were right, Kathy said, it doesn't look like Katy. They decided Katy's casket would remain closed.

Wrapped around Katy's hand was a locket from her parents. It had a four-leaf clover and a simple inscription: Mommy and Daddy.

The funeral home was jammed with family, friends, teachers, neighbors, too many people to count or remember. They came to say goodbye to Katy, but also to face their own mortality. If someone like Katy could die so young, with so much life seemingly ahead of her, it certainly proved that life is all too fragile, all too unpredictable.

Dr. Thomas Starzl walked into the funeral home, wearing a

charcoal gray suit and tie, holding on to his wife, Joy. He approached Kathy and Roger and embraced them. Starzl's wife did the same, saying little. The Millers invited Starzl to a back room.

Katy's parents had not seen Starzl since the day Katy died. Over a year and a half Starzl had formed a strong bond with Katy, and also with them. Roger on occasion snuck outside the hospital and smoked a cigar with Starzl.

Starzl always talked to the Millers about his dogs, unaware that Katy had never been an animal lover and didn't particularly like dogs. Starzl had introduced his dogs to the Millers the way parents introduce their toddlers to an old friend they encounter at the mall. *Say hi to Mrs. Miller*, Starzl told the dog when he ran into her in the parking garage at Montefiore, the dog on the front seat beside him.

Starzl also had talked to the Millers about his mother, whose death at a young age he blamed on himself. As if trying to make himself more human, he'd told them about his mother's struggle with breast cancer. He told them about the time he had to give her medicine and couldn't hold the spoon. The medicine spilled, and his mother missed a dose. He never went to church after she died, he confided.

As they sat on a couch next to the aging surgeon, the Millers looked to him for one last story, one last explanation about their daughter's death. Even in a small room with two grieving parents, Starzl found himself in the spotlight, as if there were dozens of other people with their eyes on him.

Nothing he could say would dull the heartache. The Millers wanted an unobtainable ticket to a place Starzl couldn't take them. They wanted the answers that grieving parents long for when they've lost a child, answers that still never get rid of the pain. They wanted Starzl to tell them what went wrong.

"I know there's more to it than I know," Kathy thought to herself.

On the day after Katy died, Marcos had called the Millers' house. He asked the family to come down to a meeting with the transplant team. When four of them showed up – Kathy, Roger, Shelly and Carol – they never saw Marcos. Instead, they met with Fontes, another surgeon, and Caponi, the transplant coordinator.

The surgeon explained Katy died of a cardiac arrest. Her heart had stopped beating.

"I promised her she wouldn't die," Kathy thought to herself. "I feel like a lied to her."

Starzl tried to explain what happened. *Bile ducts. Arterial lines. Portal vein. Pseudomonas.* To the Millers, however, his words turned into gibberish. They couldn't understand what Starzl was saying. Outside, there were hundreds of mourners waiting to see them and offer their sympathies. There also was a casket with their daughter inside it, and no matter what Starzl said, no matter how much thought and science he could inject into his words, nothing was going to change the outcome.

By mid-morning, the parking lot at the funeral home was clogged with cars, pickup trucks and SUVs. The Miller family sat at the front of the room, facing Katy's casket.

Kristy Miller was looking around the room when she saw a familiar face. It was Marcos. He was wearing jeans, a sports shirt and a pair of sunglasses. His Porsche was parked in the back lot. He remained in the back when the Millers' pastor began to address the crowd.

"She was only twenty-one," he said. "But in twenty-one years she probably got eighty years worth of living."

The minister spoke about Katy's fight to stay alive and the brightness of her smile. It fell to Tom Trunzo, Katy's high school principal, to inject some humor into the day. He told the story of Katy's displeasure with the new uniforms he was about to purchase for the volleyball team during her senior year.

Katy was the team captain, and Trunzo had given the young athletes several samples so they could try them on and help him make a selection. Katy barged in to his office, holding two pairs of shorts. One of them was a tight-fitting style she obviously didn't like.

"Trunzo, do you want me to play volleyball this year or not?" she asked the longtime principal at Marion Center High.

She was abrupt and sassy.

"If you think that with the size of my butt and hips, I'm going to wear those tight shorts, you are wrong," she said.

Trunzo bought the shorts Katy wanted for her team.

"I think that was an example of what she and others have informed me is the Miller attitude," Trunzo told the mourners.

One of Katy's sisters-in-law, Martina, stood up. With her husband beside her, she spoke of the time in the hospital when some relatives were playing Hangman on the white wipe-off board that hung by Katy's bed. When it was Katy's turn, she picked the word paradise.

Martina, holding on to her husband's arm, could not contain her tears. "She picked that word because that's where she should be," she said.

Martina read a poem she wrote after Katy's death. It was called "Paradise":

Since all of us knew Katy and it's so easy to see,
while she was loved by all and we all came here to be.
She had so many great qualities, it's hard to name them all;
if you needed someone to listen, she was a great one to call.
Although her personality is what won her homecoming queen,
She also had a beauty like nothing a lot of us had ever seen.
Her greatest friends in volleyball were important to her at MC,
and it's not surprising she was doing great at IUP.
Reading and watching movies is what Katy loved most, and
soaking up the sun while lying on the coast.
You could usually find her curled up with a Nora Roberts book,
But if you interrupted her, she'd just give you that look.
Katy loved getting dressed up and liked going out to dinner.
If she had a choice, Olive Garden was usually the winner.
Katy also loved her Mom's home-cooked food,
and her Dad's jokes, but only when she was in a good mood.
There are also many things Katy did not like,
And she'd be sure to tell you without putting up a fight.
Katy didn't like dogs, especially poor Tanner,
when one of them barked, you could just see her anger.
Purple, pink and hearts also did not top her list.
If a boy gave her one of these, he may have been dismissed.
Her family meant everything in the world to her,

None of us could leave without an 'I love you' and a hug, that's
for sure.
She loved playing cards with us or just our company,
When we were all together, she was as happy as can be.
Katy always had a smile on that pretty face
that nothing in this world could ever replace.
There were a lot of times she was so strong and courageous,
How she did it with so little complaint always amazed us.
Going to Ireland was Katy's dream vacation,
but it's paradise that is her final destination.
In our thoughts and prayers Katy will be, but she will surely
be missed for all eternity.

The crowd had barely had time to take in the poem when Marcos moved to the front of the room. He, too, wanted to say something. Katy's sisters looked at each other in disbelief. Shelly gripped her husband's hand. Kristy wanted to get up and stop him. *Quality of life. This will change transplantation.* Those were the words they had heard from Marcos' lips. What could he possibly say now that it was all over?

In a slow, shaky voice, Marcos said he'd given many speeches in his life but didn't know what quite to say now. He spoke about Linton Guadalupe, the man he cared for in a Venezuelan hospital. He never gave Linton's age, but Marcos said the two became fast friends while the man was treated for gastric cancer.

"I became so attached to this patient, I used to change his dressings three times a day," Marcos said. He pushed his wheelchair, and they smoked cigarettes outside the hospital. They forged a bond that even Marcos knew was wrong.

"We can never cross the line," he said. "We as doctors take care of patients. We can never be so involved with them as if it were your family."

Marcos thought he'd learned his lesson until he met Katy.

"I have to say today I've crossed that line again with Katy," he said.

Marcos' words seemed genuine, thoughtful, deliberate. As he spoke, Starzl never looked up. He didn't want to cross eyes with the man with whom he'd struggled to forge a professional bond, the man who was supposed to help him change organ transplantation. Starzl had dedicated a lifetime to the creation of Katy's immunosuppressive protocol. Her death was the protocol's death. She was about to be buried, along with the promise of a renaissance for a field that was stagnant at best.

Starzl had said many times he had never had a personal bond or connection with Marcos. They had been polar opposites, brought together by science and medicine and the power that can come along with it.

Starzl's eyes fixed on Katy's casket and the cascade of white roses that covered it. Then he heard Marcos' words.

"I think I lost my daughter today," Marcos told the group. "There's nothing that I can tell you that will make the pain go away, and I wish I would have been able to help."

I don't know what Starzl was thinking, but it was clear by his actions in the previous year that he thought Marcos should have been more honest about Katy's case. There was no need to point fingers or to make accusations. Science wasn't like that. Starzl knew full well that death is inevitable. He knew full well that medicine always had been ripe for setbacks and obstacles. He'd told me so in one of our interviews, when I asked him about transplantation's derailment into a business, rather than the crusade Starzl had launched.

"The worries have always been there since the beginning because of the act of taking a piece of somebody's body and making it survive in somebody else's body, from the dawn of time, has had all kinds of abuse and misapplications," he'd told me.

Starzl had invoked Leonardo Da Vinci to justify the risks artists – and scientists – must take to achieve their creations. He told me how Da Vinci had robbed graves so he could dissect bodies and draw what he had found. And he told me how success, even in a field as life-saving and life-changing as organ transplantation, breeds trouble.

"By and large, with the commercialization of anything, and specifically organ transplantation all over the world, people are very concerned about brokering organ sales and, you know, in India and all these places, abuses are everywhere," he said. "There's a lot to worry about. And yet there is so much benefit. I think at a practical level transplantation really is one of the great advances of the 20th century in medicine overall."

When he spoke about the success of transplantation, Starzl late in his life became keenly aware of it as a field that had been commercialized. Perhaps Marcos, standing at the funeral home before him, had helped to foster that notion. Transplant volume shot up when Marcos arrived at UPMC. His predecessor had been ordered to keep an eye on volume.

"I actually have never been interested in the money, ever," Starzl said. "Making money from transplantation was never even a priority at all, much less a high one."

Starzl had always realized the larger-than-life implications of transplantation. The surgery was huge, he'd told me once. Yet as he watched Katy's casket, it was as if all those years of labor had gone to waste. *Layers of grief.* Starzl had reached a point in his life where those layers were too thick to withstand.

As the service concluded, Starzl watched as Katy's four brothers and three sisters surrounded the casket. They touched it, hoping the touch of cold metal could make them closer to Katy one last time. They lifted the casket and slowly walked out of the funeral home. They walked past Marcos, who stood by the door with a solemn face.

Marcos smiled at Kristy. It seemed like a half-smirk that felt invasive. *He had the audacity to smile*, she'd tell me later. *Douche bag.* Katy's illness caused her family to carry a weight so heavy that by the time she died, few of her brothers and sisters had the strength to carry it. Kristy was one of them, and Marcos' presence felt like a bug crawling under her skin, she said. His presence was a reminder that her healing, and that of her family's, would take a long time to occur, if it ever happened.

After it became clear that Katy's first transplant had failed, Kristy had not been able to hide her emotions, even in front of Katy. She was sitting at her parents' home one evening, crying on the couch, when Katy walked in.

"What's the matter?" Katy asked.

"I don't want you to die," Kristy told her, unable to conceal the pain that comes with knowing that your young sister is seriously ill.

"I'm not going to die," Katy promised. "This isn't going to beat me."

12

Banished

Thomas Starzl always thought big. Katy's death pushed him to think bigger. He wanted the world to know what had happened. He wanted everyone to know that complications in live-donor liver transplants were higher than ever reported.

In the months after Katy's death, he worked furiously to craft a paper about his findings: significant complications in just about two-thirds of patients.

Aiming to get the biggest bang for his buck, Starzl in October 2007 submitted his findings to the prestigious New England Journal of Medicine.

His bosses at the University of Pittsburgh scoffed at his strategy. Telling the world via such a widely regarded scientific journal that their program had complication rates higher than reported elsewhere would be devastating.

Ten days after Starzl submitted the paper, Dr. Timothy Billiar, chairman of surgery, wrote to Starzl. In an unprecedented move, Billiar asked him to withdraw the manuscript.

At the same time, Dr. Arthur S. Levine, the senior vice chancellor for health sciences and dean of the medical school, dashed off a two-paragraph email to the editor of the journal, Jeffrey M. Drazen.

Levine point-blank asked Drazen to stop the paper from publication.

"My colleagues and I perceive very substantial problems with this report," Levine wrote. "The problems we have identified focus on the requirements of HIPAA; appropriate authorship designation; the quality of the patient data assembled and presented; and the interpretation of those data."

Levine didn't stop there. He admitted that Starzl's standing in the university – and in the world's scientific community – made the problem all the more difficult. "Given Dr. Starzl's great stature in the medical and scientific communities, dealing with this manuscript has been a painful exercise," he wrote.

Five days later, Levine wrote a more detailed letter to Drazen, this time around making a more dramatic plea. "The manuscript is a simple description of the results of one surgeon's patients without hypothesis or context." The surgeon wasn't mentioned by name in the letter. It was Marcos. "The single surgeon is not a co-author, did not participate in the analysis, and does not approve of the submission."

Levine told Drazen that Starzl's analysis was premature and incomplete. The plea worked. The paper was not published.

Starzl was livid. People throughout his career may have questioned him, but no one ever dared undermine him. He was certain that the rate of complications that had been reported by Marcos and others was much lower than the data showed. As far as he was concerned, the truth needed to get out.

Tensions escalated between Starzl and administrators. On Oct. 23, 2007, Billiar issued a terse memo to the transplant institute's faculty. Although it was addressed to the "Starzl Transplantation Institute Faculty," the fact that the word Starzl was part of the institute's name appeared to mean nothing.

Billiar made it clear that "Starzl does not meet the criteria for being provided with access to protected health information." He urged faculty to not provide protected health information to anyone unless they were directly involved in the care of the patient or were an investigator named in a protocol approved by the university's Institutional Review Board. "This restriction includes Dr. Starzl," Billiar wrote.

It was a clear and unyielding directive. Starzl's credentials and reputation be damned. No name was big enough to get in the way of the university's powerful leaders. Starzl fired back several times, at one point telling one UPMC administrator that he was not violating patient privacy laws.

It didn't matter. On November 16, Starzl received a letter at his home, minutes away from the institute that bore his name. It was signed by John Innocenti, president of UPMC Presbyterian and Montefiore hospitals and John Houston, UPMC's security chief.

"Although it is with considerable regret given your long association with UPMC...we are compelled to inform you that you are not permitted in any UPMC facilities, except in the limited case where you

need to receive medical care."

Starzl had been banned from setting foot at the hospital where he'd pioneered liver transplant surgery.

I learned that administrators in those days were so disillusioned with Starzl, they attributed it to senility and aging. But I knew better. Starzl was filled with indignation. Now, he had nowhere to turn.

□ ❑ □ ❑ □ ❑ □

It was mid-morning when we arrived at Starzl's office, and it didn't take long to feel the tension in the air. My colleague Andy Conte and I walked through a dirty glass door and up the steps into the narrow maze of hallways.

Starzl's dogs greeted us with loud barks. They provided a rudimentary security service in an office that seemed ill-fitted for a man of Starzl's stature. The carpet was torn, the walls scuffed, the metal furniture rusted.

The building, along a busy road perpetually clogged with traffic, was far from the offices of the most prominent scientists at UPMC. Is this what Starzl wanted, or is this what the upper brass thought he was worth?

Starzl appeared wearing a dark suit, mumbling something to his assistant, Terry Mangan. He seemed jittery, but greeted us with affection and respect.

"We can't meet in my office," he said. "I think it's better if we meet in a different room."

He ushered us into a small room with two worn couches. There were no pictures on the walls and no fancy decorations.

"This is better," he said. "No one can hear us here."

Starzl, or at the very least someone in his staff, was afraid his third-floor office was bugged. He believed the higher-ups at the university, intent on finding out what he was talking about to the press, had somehow installed a listening device in his office. Although the level of paranoia seemed unusual and hyperbolic, I wasn't entirely surprised. Starzl, after all, had been banned from the transplant institute named after him. After Katy's death, he created a tidal wave of controversy and was loud enough for the upper tier of UPMC bosses to pay attention.

Katy had been his star patient, the key to an unblemished legacy. Once she got a new liver, she wasn't supposed to get sick. She was supposed to progress, grow old and soar. When Katy grew sick again, Starzl became obsessed with trying to figure out why.

That first meeting with him, in February 2008, wasn't meant to be about Katy. Instead, we wanted to hear Starzl's views about a practice occurring in transplant centers in the United States: Surgeons who were transplanting livers in hundreds of patients who didn't need the surgery. Over a four-month period, we had discovered that four transplant centers in the country – including UPMC – topped the list of hospitals doing the surgeries.

The practice was the opposite of Starzl's deeply held belief that scarce livers should first be offered to the sickest patients.

But using federally sanctioned data from UNOS, we found that people at the bottom of the wait list were getting new livers even though they stood to live longer without it.

Our story was scheduled to run in several weeks, and we needed Starzl's reaction. We knew he was opposed to the practice, and we needed him to tell us so.

It wasn't easy to do. For one, Starzl wasn't alone during the interview. Sitting inches away from him was Randy Juhl, a former pharmacy school dean turned vice chancellor for research and compliance. It was obvious Starzl and Juhl liked each other, but Starzl wanted to play mind games.

He told us he would have preferred to meet with us alone. He referred to Juhl as a chaperone, sent by UPMC officials who were worried about what Starzl would say.

"I'm offended by the fact that they can't drop by and say hello without having a custodian without otherwise creating a crisis here," Starzl said, referring to us. "It's really amazing to me."

"If you want, I'm happy to leave," Juhl said.

"I'd just as soon have you stay."

The back-and-forth stretched for nearly two hours. It took a lot of heavy lifting to get answers out of Starzl. He complained about a photographer who was taking his picture, convinced that the photographer planned to ignore his request to be photographed alongside Juhl.

"I just have to have your word that you are not going to take a picture of us and snip off half," he asked.

It was all part of the Starzl act. He wanted to show UPMC that he wasn't straying too far from what they wanted. He may have been the father of transplantation, but he still answered to university officials. He needed to abide by their rules.

But Starzl knew better. He knew that he could speak his own mind, even with Juhl sitting two feet away. Starzl finally delivered: Yes, he believed in the "sickest first" principle to dole out organs. That was the Pittsburgh position and worldwide position, he said, to always give preference to the sickest patients. Bingo. He said it, regardless if the room was bugged or not, and in the presence of a top university official.

"There are transplants being done that shouldn't be done," he said. "You are going to the extreme end of replacing the engine, when maybe all you have to do is do a spark plug."

If he thought anyone was listening, Starzl made sure his words stung. He delivered a strong jab to Marcos, when I told him that Marcos, in an interview, said he wanted Pittsburgh to remain a mecca of organ transplantation.

"That's a very candid commercial statement," Starzl said about Marcos. "I mean, you know, this is not a football game, where you are trying to run up the score."

Because there had been a shift in philosophy, I asked if he was worried about his legacy. Starzl became testy.

"I think it would be a shallow point of view to suggest that my legacy depends on Pittsburgh," he said. "I would think that would be pretty shortsighted."

The way he saw it, organ transplantation didn't necessarily start in Pittsburgh, but rather at the University of Colorado, where he'd begun his career. Even so, Starzl made it clear he believed understanding the immune system was by all means much more important than performing the actual transplant surgery. Despite his big words and lengthy answers, Starzl seemed to be in favor of the truth.

"I come from a family of journalists," he said, in obvious reference to his father, Rome, who had been owner of a semiweekly newspaper in Iowa. His uncle, Frank, had been general manager for The Associated Press in New York. "And I believe that journalists are highly moral people, and that good journalists put out material that is at least as accurate as what you find in scientific journals. It's quite a bit more understandable, but it's at least as accurate."

Almost without warning, the conversation shifted to Katy.

He didn't have to say it, but I knew the Katy Miller protocol had consumed the recent years of Starzl's life. Pieced together, his entire career and its many chapters had been devoted to crafting the right answer to the question of tolerance.

Yet Starzl was enamored with much more than science. Whether he admitted it or not, he was bewitched by his patients. He was entranced by their illnesses and their ability to fight hard against them. If he became attached to them, it was because he was attached to what they represented and what they could contribute to the future of medicine. Like other patients he had nurtured and treated, Katy personified the science that so defined Starzl. Every time she smiled, science was smiling at him, too.

"I've never actually seen such an outpouring of grief," he said about her death.

Andy, my colleague, asked him if Katy's case changed his relationship with Marcos.

"I think it changed my relationship to everything," he said.

Then he mentioned Stormie Jones. She was the 7-year-old Texas girl who made medical history when she became the world's first person to receive simultaneous liver and heart transplants. She died of heart rejection in 1990 at age 13.

Starzl, who had his own heart problems that year, decided he couldn't take care of patients anymore.

"Grief is like that," he said. "Your mother dies, or some particular patient dies, these are devastating hits. And you know, in the course of a long and tough life doing difficult cases and being always right at the edge of tertiary care problems, you build up layers of grief. But you can take those if they are thin. But when you have a deep rip in the fabric, that's a different matter. And Katy was like that."

Two months later, in April 2008, Marcos resigned from UPMC. It was an abrupt departure for a man who had been so widely portrayed by administrators as the new transplant king. In a brief phone conversation, Marcos told me his exit had nothing to do with Starzl's findings. When I asked why complications in live-donor liver transplants were higher than in transplants using dead donors, he said: "That's to be expected." He reminded me that few people die as a result of those complications.

"I have done this surgery more times than anyone else in this country," he said. "I intend to keep on doing them."

But his Pittburgh chapter was over and so was the protocol, halted after his departure.

In November 2008, Andy and I once again met with Starzl and Juhl. Our stories about liver transplants on people who would not benefit from them had already been published, a three-part series titled "Transplanting Too Soon." Impressive work, Starzl told me about the series in a phone conversation.

Two days before that meeting, we'd also published a story about his review of live-donor liver transplant complications, based in part on an interview we'd done with Dr. Wallis Marsh, who was appointed interim chief of transplantation upon Marcos' departure. Starzl often called him Wally, a nickname Marsh didn't like. But it was Starzl, and you had to take anything he called you.

Starzl, who had been outside the United States, and thus unable to be interviewed, finally agreed to talk about the issue. This time around, we met in Juhl's office at the Cathedral of Learning, a 42-story building where the university's administrative offices are located. It was a rainy day and, having no umbrellas, we walked in to Juhl's office quite wet.

We were eager to confront Starzl about the New England Journal paper – the one the medical school dean yanked from publication.

Juhl decorated his office with odd-shaped glass bottles filled with brightly colored liquids. We sat at a long, wooden table facing Starzl and Juhl. Starzl seemed small and frail, and stroked a folder whose contents he never revealed. Almost as if Starzl weren't in the room, Juhl told us how the father of transplantation beat himself up over his failures.

"What has kept Dr. Starzl at the forefront all these years is to look at the failures," he said. "We pat ourselves on the back for our successes, but where we move the science ahead is to look at the ones who didn't do well and say, well, why not? Let me fix that. That really is the next step of the scientific part."

All Starzl wanted to do was make things better, Juhl reasoned, using the kind of academic tone I'm sure many of his students found dense and lackadaisical. The conversation stretched for nearly two hours, but it took a lot of work to get answers out of Starzl. There's no real reason to ask my opinion, he said at one point.

He didn't want to talk about a chapter of his life that caused so much heartache and professional turmoil. He was, by his own admission, way past retirement age. At 80, he should have been at home listening to his favorite Mozart tunes, not worrying about the effects of immunosuppression on the human body.

"I haven't been seeing patients for almost 20 years," Starzl told us. "So, normally, I hardly even go to the hospital."

Yet Starzl and Juhl explained how Starzl became concerned about the rate of complications and was eager to figure out if they were a result of the surgery – or what happened *after* the surgery.

Juhl downplayed the feud between Starzl and the transplant center administrators, and I was peeved. Scientists argue, much in the same way journalists argue with editors, he told us, using an analogy he thought we'd find understandable. Sometimes those arguments get heated and really personal, but that was as much as he would say. He wanted to move on from the subject, and we wouldn't let him.

I recited a litany of transgressions against Starzl: that he wasn't allowed to step into the transplant center named after him, that the dean of the medical school sent a letter to the New England Journal of Medicine to discredit his research and so on.

"Those are pretty serious steps to be taken by these parties in connection with a person of the stature of Dr. Starzl," I said. "So obviously there has to be some reaction to that kind of behavior."

Silence filled the room.

"I think in retrospect there are a lot of things that occurred that would not qualify for work in the diplomatic corps," Juhl conceded, but it was obvious he was growing uncomfortable with the questions.

Is he allowed to go into the Starzl Institute now and go into the hospital? I pushed.

The two are different places, Juhl replied, as if I didn't know. "But when you were prohibited from entering any premises, what were the places that you were..." I said before Starzl interrupted me.

"Let's see," he said.

"He didn't pay attention to any of this," Juhl said.

"Are you prohibited now from going to Montefiore or going in to meet patients?" I asked.

"No, I'm not."

"Were you at one point?"

"Well, I suppose," Starzl said. "I think it was a clerical error."

"What kind of a clerical error?" I said, knowing full well that no clerical error would result in the banishment of a scientific icon from a center named after him.

"It's really sort of too complicated, and I'm not offended by it by the way."

"By?"

"By what happened," Starzl said. "It was a cleansing process. Do you think?"

"Yeah," Juhl said.

"On whose part?"

"Maybe on everybody's part," Starzl said. "I think we had a boat that had a hole in it and required fixing that hole."

Starzl remained painfully stubborn for most of the conversation, often telling us we already had the answers to our questions.

"You had it pretty straight in the paper, in your article," Starzl said. "Your article was very precise."

But why had he become so involved, so mesmerized by this matter? Had it been because the high rate of complications could give a black eye to the field he'd created? Had it been because he wanted to expose Marcos and his failure to accurately report the complications? Or had it been Katy, whose own case had been marred by management oversights?

Juhl, along with University of Pittsburgh Chancellor Mark Nordenberg, painstakingly ironed out the differences between Starzl and hospital administrators. All agreed the solution rested on a brand new, independent review of the complications, this time led by Marsh, a trusted and savvy surgeon, in collaboration with Starzl, his mentor in the 1980s.

To accurately examine complications, the men used a scale developed in 2004 by Dr. Pierre-Alain Clavien, a Swiss transplant surgeon. The Clavien method categorized surgical complications from minor infections to death, according to their severity.

"That's the beauty of the Clavien system, and that's why you can't conceal complications if you use the Clavien system," Starzl said. "It's a very objective system."

As Starzl put it, no one in the world had looked at complications with such purpose, with such a detailed eye. He wanted the truth – the true rate, as he explained, sometimes staring at the table or directly at Juhl, looking for his silent approval.

In his earlier review of the 126 Pittsburgh cases, Starzl found that more than 60 percent of the recipients experienced a complication that required another medical intervention. Many of them were bile duct leaks. The complications weren't easy to conceal. They were there, in black and white on the medical records and operating room records, easy for Starzl to find.

The new review was nearly identical. With five cases tossed for technical reasons, it zeroed in on 121 cases strictly of right-lobe liver transplantation, the most common form of the surgery. The surgeons, with the help of statisticians, tagged nearly two-thirds – 79 cases – of the cases with the label Clavien III or higher. Those patients, they noted, had required a medical intervention such as a second surgery following the transplant.

The Clavien system identified the complication by virtue of that follow-up treatment or surgery, Starzl explained.

"If I gave you a liver, and it required an operation later, automatically that's a complication," he said. "And it's identified as such by virtue of the fact that it had to be treated."

About 41 percent of the reviewed cases involved patients who experienced biliary leaks or blockages. The leaks – when bile collects outside the bile ducts – can correct themselves, but can be life-threatening. They can require surgical repair. In addition, the review found 15 percent of patients experienced vascular complications; 9 percent experienced other issues.

Plain and simple, Starzl said, the rate of complications was "higher than reported elsewhere."

"It may be that complications are being underreported elsewhere," he said. "Knowing surgeons as I do, that would be a natural expectation, to underestimate."

An earlier study, in October 2008, by a federally sanctioned group known as the Adult-to-Adult Living Donor Liver Transplantation Cohort Study, presented quite different findings. Supported by the National Institutes of Health, the study reported a 42 percent rate of all types and degrees of bile duct leakage and blockage among live donor liver transplant recipients. It used a 1994 version of the Clavien scale.

Knowing that we were on to a big story, Starzl asked us to be careful in the way we delivered our message to newspaper readers.

"It has to be delivered in a very subtle way because we don't want to be out there saying everybody is lying," he said.

I left the meeting thinking about lies. In many ways I was pleased Starzl had spoken his mind. He finally had freed himself from the corporate muzzle that stopped him from telling the truth.

As I walked out with Andy in the afternoon drizzle, I remembered a morning several months earlier in which I'd shown up at Starzl's office. I'd heard he'd submitted his first review on transplant complications to the New England Journal. Starzl denied such a paper existed.

"I don't know what you are talking about," he told me as he sat next to Terry Mangan, his assistant.

I had a feeling he wasn't telling the truth, but I left, convinced that people often have little choice but to be duplicitous. Surely he's on the trail of a higher truth, and it's a road that's littered with denials and falsehoods, I told myself.

"I didn't really lie to you, but I didn't fork over the full story at the time," he'd told me in the November meeting with Juhl.

I was OK with it. He was fighting for Katy's honor.

13

Layers of grief

Every night before going to bed, Thomas Starzl's wife got on her knees and prayed.

Joy Starzl prayed before every meal, and pretty much anytime she could.

"She never has a meal without saying a prayer," Starzl told me in October 2010 during one of our many unplanned, often brief, but always meaningful telephone conversations. "It's reassuring at times."

I had called Starzl to ask a few questions about jaundice – the yellowing of the skin as a result of liver trouble. In his book, he had described it as a lemon or orange hue caused by bile that can't be discharged and that accumulates in the bloodstream. No sooner had I asked about it, than I found myself talking about religion instead of medicine. It wasn't at all strange for this to happen – to begin a conversation about one subject and jump to another without warning.

He'd done the same many times before when my question about

academia or immunology turned into a 10-minute discourse on movies, his liking of President Obama or professional football. One memorable morning, Starzl called my office, promptly returning a call, and I asked if he'd watched Super Bowl XL. The night before, on Feb. 5, 2006, the Pittsburgh Steelers had just defeated the Seattle Seahawks.

"I don't believe we've had a chance to discuss the Steelers victory," Starzl told me. For the next ten minutes, he discussed interceptions, turnovers and blown calls with the same air of authority he spoke about anatomy and the biliary system.

The chat about religion was a first, and one that I particularly was eager to have in light of Katy's case. Would her death cause Starzl to change? Would he become a more spiritual man? *You build up layers of grief. Life is full of devastating hits.*

Spirituality always has been part of medicine but it's most often been the patients who speak about finding prayer and spiritual direction as a result of a medical encounter. Patients crave the reassurance that the person who is treating them not only knows what he's doing but has the capability to restore their health no matter what.

Every surgeon, every doctor I've ever talked to about the subject of spirituality has admitted that some patients view them as a higher power. It's not that the doctors considered themselves superhuman; it was just that other people did. Rightfully or not, doctors are seen by the populace as godlike because of their power to heal.

"You tell patients they can die on the operating room table, and they put their faith in you," one of Katy's surgeons, Ngoc Thai, told me. "You're asking them to stare at the face of death."

I doubt Starzl considered himself God, but many of his former patients praised his godlike wisdom to fight nature and fix a medical problem so complex it seemed almost impossible to conquer.

"I always call him the angel on my shoulder," Betty Baird told me. She was one of Starzl's first liver transplant patients in 1979, when he was doing experimental surgeries in Colorado. "I love him to death."

When Starzl mentioned his wife's propensity to prayer, I immediately asked him if he prayed, hoping to hear him say that he had prayed for Katy. *How could he not?* I told myself. *How can Starzl, having been involved in more than 10,000 transplant surgeries, not have prayed for any of his patients, especially those who didn't make it?*

His answer was blunt, the way he was about pretty much everything.

"I don't pray," he said. "But I admire those who do."

"Are you spiritual?" I asked, wanting more specifics. Journalists don't like generalities.

"Yes, but not within the confines of a denomination," Starzl said.

His answer came as no surprise. Even though Starzl had been a Latin scholar and once considered becoming a priest, he stopped going to church after his mother's funeral Mass. Twenty-nine years passed before he set foot in a church again, to pay respects to his father.

"I go to church from time to time," he said. His wife practiced her faith at a Baptist church, which often exposed Starzl to lively services rich with music and passion. "They celebrate momentary freedom from poverty. I enjoy taking Joy because of it."

Joy Starzl was a black woman in a white man's world, the unlikely wife of a powerful medical icon. Starzl met the former Joy Conger in 1977, when he was biking to the University of Colorado General Hospital. Joy, on her way to work as a lab technician, hit him with her car. He told her he was OK and, a week later, they went out to lunch in what became a series of regular dates. During those early days of courtship, Starzl never told Joy he was a surgeon.

Once they married, it was Joy who reminded Starzl there was a higher power looking after him, his family and his patients. That became apparent when Starzl had a health scare while performing liver transplant surgery on Christmas Eve 1986. He was at Children's Hospital of Pittsburgh, and the patient was an infant who was bleeding because his blood would not clot. Starzl was using an instrument to dry up tissue when he burned the back of his left eye. He could only see with one eye. The trouble was only temporary, but Joy reacted in a way that surprised Starzl, according to his memoir.

"Thank you, Jesus," she said when he came home from the emergency room.

He was befuddled by such a response, but she clarified: "This means you won't have to work so hard."

I tried to ask him questions about this incident during our phone conversation, but Starzl wanted no part of it. He was spent.

"You are sucking me dry," he said before hanging up.

Yes, Tom Starzl was a tired man but he was a man with a mission. The field he built had morphed into something he almost didn't recognize. While his mantra had always been to first treat the very sick, surgeons were now putting new livers in patients who were seemingly healthy, able to play golf, shop at the mall or swim at the pool.

During one of our conversations, Starzl told me about his involvement in the transplantation council that set up federal rules for organ allocation.

"It met periodically and one of the questions that kept coming up at that meeting was what should our position be about organ allocation?" Starzl said. "Basically the rules for organ allocation that are in place today in the United States of America were all written here in Pittsburgh."

He spoke about those days with the memory of someone much younger. He recited names of medical journals and meetings way in the past. *Sickest first*. That was the mantra of the field, and everyone agreed – surgeons and hospital administrators in Pittsburgh and across the United States.

The shift in philosophy, subtle to the average person but so clear to him, seemed unreal, preposterous, obscene. Sickest first, because there is no other option, he told me.

"That is the ruling principle…that's the Pittsburgh position," he'd told me. "And it has become now the worldwide position."

Starzl believed that patients should not be treated by a physician the way a warden would treat inmates in a penitentiary. A physician's obligation, if at all possible, was to develop a collaborative approach to care.

"The ultimate objective if at all possible should be to liberate the patient from control of the physician rather than to exercise control," he said. "That means that almost every major decision starting with the decision for or against transplantation, even decisions about medications, should be made in collaboration with patients."

As he saw it, when physicians chose to replace the whole engine – as with a liver transplant – they were obligated to take into account not statistics, but rather the patient's wishes. Ultimately, it would be a decision about the quality of their lives.

Had Katy's wishes been considered throughout her illness? Or was she talked into a transplant that she could have waited for?

As he aged, with conference centers, buildings and even a street named after him on the campus of the University of Pittsburgh, Starzl steamed at the thought of organ transplantation morphing into a business. From crusade to business, that's how he explained it.

Walt Disney, Edward R. Murrow, Bill Gates, all of them began their careers with a discovery and made tremendous impact, he said.

"But if you have an impact, you have to have a delivery system that involves capitalism," Starzl said.

Starzl learned about capitalism from John Bogle, a Wall Street insider who founded Vanguard Group, one of the largest mutual funds in the world. Bogle was as skilled in money matters as Starzl was in medicine. *Time* magazine named him one of the world's most powerful and influential people.

When Bogle wrote about the apparently deceptive workings of the finance world, it resonated with Starzl. Bogle wrote about greedy investors lining their own pockets while everyone else suffered. Starzl wanted me to read the book, and I knew why. In much the same way

Bogle indicted corporate America, Starzl believed the business and ethical standards of medicine had been compromised.

"That's been called the fight for the soul of the university," he said in obvious reference to Bogle's book, *The Battle for the Soul of Capitalism.*"

Starzl's own battle reached a denouement when he told me in February 2008 he wanted to retire.

"I have battle fatigue," he told me. "I want out the door of involvement in transplantation."

Starzl had spent his last days closing up his research work, sorting through boxes and filing cabinets stuffed with dusty journals and yellowed papers. In a move replete with irony, he sold his collection of scientific papers to the University of Pittsburgh for $1.

Katy's case had drained him. *Grief is like that.* He talked to his old protégé, John Fung, who had moved on to the Cleveland Clinic, and the two friends spoke about the rate of complications in live donor surgeries; about Marcos and his quest to build an empire; about the inevitable commercialization of the surgery he had perfected.

"You shouldn't be involved with any of this stuff," Fung told him. "Just give your lectures, you know, enjoy life."

Fung, like many others who had spoken to Starzl in the past few months, worried about the surgeon's health.

"It's so draining on him, energy-wise, he looks so tired," Fung told me when I met him at his Cleveland office to talk about the newspaper article about early liver transplants on people who don't need zthem. "I don't think he's eating well. I don't think he's taking care of himself, and it's all this stress, what can I do? I tell him he should take it easy, don't do it. And he still does it anyway."

Starzl hesitated only momentarily when my colleague, Andy Conte, and I asked the obligatory question about his legacy.

"I never did have a big game plan," he said. "If you don't have a big game plan, then you really don't have something that you strive for and accomplish and have as your cherished legacy. I just came to work and did the best I could. I behaved myself. I never got arrested. I don't even have a misdemeanor on my record, and I'm proud of that. So I suppose that's my legacy."

Talking about an arrest, hardly the image conjured up when talking about a half-century career in operating rooms and hospital corridors, was a deliberate allusion to a little-known arrest of Amadeo Marcos. The surgeon who operated on Katy had been arrested by the Pittsburgh police in June 2007 on a charge of simple assault.

Police records stated that Marcos and a female passenger were arguing loudly in his silver Porsche Cayenne. Marcos pressed the woman against the passenger door. Her lip was cut and bleeding. She told police Marcos punched her four or five times in the face and head because he had asked her to get out of the car and she wouldn't. The left side of her head was red and swollen. Marcos told police they were arguing because she wouldn't give back his car keys.

Although the incident happened in June, the police report didn't surface for nearly eight months. I tried to contact the woman, whose name was on the police documents. She'd told police she was in an ongoing intimate relationship with Marcos, who was married to another physician.

I found her on Myspace.com. I was surprised at her quick response and her candor, even after I identified myself as a newspaper reporter. *We are close friends,* she told me, referring to Marcos. She'd chosen not to press charges as long as Marcos followed through with an order to enroll in an eight-session anger-management program.

My editor at the time, the late Bob Fryer, made the decision to not report the arrest. Not only was the report eight months old, it also was unknown if it was related to Marcos' sudden departure from the university in March 2008. The independent study of complications in Marcos' liver transplant surgeries seemed like a more plausible explanation for his departure, even if administrators were unwilling to admit it.

Marcos never spoke about what happened. He never answered my repeated calls or responded to a letter I left at his house. I called him so much to talk about Katy that one colleague urged me to stop, concerned that Marcos would think I was harassing him.

Before he left UPMC, Marcos met with us several times to answer questions about unnecessary transplants. He said he never used organs from unsuitable donors.

"Nobody in his right mind would do a transplant not expecting for it to succeed," he said. "You're not going to take an organ for somebody's that's desperate when you know it's going to fail. That doesn't happen."

Starzl's words belied the influence the Marcos debacle had on him. *I never got arrested.* Had Starzl's career been diluted to one moment, one case, one person? Katy. *Grief is like that.*

If Starzl had been transformed, so had the field of organ

transplantation – at least from the standpoint of the amount and type of surgeries that still were being done. The surgeries using live-donors took a particularly devastating hit in 2010 with the deaths of two men who donated part of their livers to their sick relatives. The deaths, at the Lahey Clinic near Boston and the University of Colorado Hospital, prompted the programs to be temporarily suspended as surgeons once again debated the advantages of risking the life of a healthy donor.

The deaths would not deter Dr. Abhinav Humar, who arrived in Pittsburgh from the University of Minnesota in 2009 to replace Marcos. Humar said the two cases, which were not tied to the quality of care at either of the two centers, would cause him to be more vigilant about the surgeries, but they would continue.

"The right approach is not to bury your head in the sand and say that this can't happen," Humar told me at the time. "That risk is there. Donors are better served knowing all the potential risks and complications so they can make an informed decision."

Then in 2011, the Pittsburgh transplant program took another hit. Administrators in May of that year disclosed surgeons transplanted a kidney from a donor infected with the hepatitis C virus. They said a nurse and a surgeon overlooked a patient chart that contained information about the infection. Administrators voluntarily suspended the live-donor kidney transplant programs, as well as the live-donor liver transplant program. The case, unknown to the public until the *Pittsburgh Tribune-Review* broke the story, became front-page news in Pittsburgh as UPMC officials struggled to contain the public relations damage. Some patients abandoned UPMC, choosing instead to get listed with a fledgling program at rival

Allegheny General Hospital. Federal reviewers from UNOS eventually blamed human error for the oversight. UPMC administrators apologized and reopened the program two months later.

Starzl never made any public comments about the hepatitis C case. I called him several times, trying to get him to talk about it. He was a smart man and didn't want to tarnish his name by linking it to a story that was far removed from anything he had ever accomplished.

"I haven't talked to anyone in Pittsburgh in over a week," he told me one day. He was speaking on his cell phone, and I could hear noise in the background. He was at the Denver airport, on his way back to Pittsburgh.

I reminded him to call me back. I had developed enough rapport with Starzl that I felt comfortable enough to protest when he didn't return a phone call. One time he mentioned the August 2010 wedding of his grandson, Ravi, to a UPMC nurse. I jokingly wondered why I had not received an invitation. Two days later I received in the mail a beautiful, engraved invitation to the wedding at The Grand Hall at The Priory in Pittsburgh. A previous commitment prevented me from attending.

Starzl had continued his relationship with Katy Miller's family, but only for the first year after her death. He showed up with Joy and several of his dogs at a memorial walk in Indiana, Pennsylvania, held in Katy's honor. He strolled around for several miles and asked Kathy and Roger general questions about the family. It was hard for Starzl to look into the eyes of Roger Miller; Starzl had lost a patient, but Roger had lost a daughter. When Starzl left, he told Kathy he'd see her next year. He'd be back, he said. But he never did return. *Grief is like that.*

In my many conversations with Kathy, she always asked about Starzl. *Have you spoken to him? How is he doing?* Starzl was a link to Katy, and Kathy did not want those ties to be severed. He was a reminder of everything that had happened and everything that *could have* happened. It didn't matter that seeing him, or even thinking about Starzl, transported her back to UPMC, right there in the room with Katy, watching her yellow skin, watching her die.

When I called Kathy, I always felt I was reopening old wounds by bringing up Katy. I asked questions about what Katy ate when she was sick, what she wore to doctor's appointments, what class she was taking when she got sick. Kathy never grew tired of my questions. It was the reverse: She yearned to relive her daughter's life. She yearned to talk about her, to think about her and to imagine her talk, her smell, her beauty.

"There's not a day that goes by that I don't think about her."

One summer day, she drove me to Katy's grave. She jumped in her car, and I followed her. *Isn't it nice?* she asked, and what can you say when someone poses that question before their daughter's grave? She smiled faintly, as if trying to diminish her grief. There is no timetable for grief, however deep it is inside you.

For a few minutes, we took in the peace and quiet. I felt helpless watching Kathy. *Why does grief hurt so much? Why can't we go back to what once was?* When I noticed Kathy's eyes well with tears, I cried, too, unable to shake off the numb feeling that takes over when you're surrounded by death, trying to find answers to those questions.

It took almost three years for me to find anything that resembled an answer. It was in the summer of 2011, at a golf outing Katy's family held every year to honor her memory.

I was expecting only a few people, but was surprised to find the Meadow Lane Golf Course in Indiana packed with young golfers. Just before they set out to golf, the group gathered under a pavilion where Katy's sisters set up a table with photographs of Katy. Many of the guys stopped by, picked up the photo albums and smiled as they flipped through the images – Katy in her volleyball uniform, at the beach with Shelly, and at her 21st birthday party, her skin so yellow that the photo looked like there was something wrong with the paper.

A little girl named Katya ran around the pavilion, her brown hair bunched in pigtails. Katya was the daughter of Martina and Josh, one of Katy's twin brothers. Katy never met Katya; she died in the days when Josh and Martina found out they were expecting. The couple asked Katy's parents if they could name the baby after Katy. Kathy told them there was only one Katy, but agreed to their idea of adding an "a" to form the name Katya.

Several days before the golf outing, Katya and her grandmother, Kathy, spent time on the swing set in the Millers' backyard. The golf event was looming and Kathy wanted to talk about it, even if it was with a three-year-old.

"Is Katy going to be at the golf outing?" Katya asked.

"No, honey, she won't be there."

"Why not?"

"She was sick and she had to go to heaven," Kathy said, holding back tears.

"Oh, I wanted to play with her," Katya said. "I wanted to see her."

Grandmother and granddaughter remained quiet for several minutes, until Katya pointed to the bright blue sky above her.

"See that cloud?" she told her grandma. "Katy's up there."

Final Word

ABOUT ME ◆ By Katy Miller

I love to read and get lost in a world that no one can ruin +

I love soft lips and rough hands ;) +

I respect those who have standards and morals and those who are honest and truthful (even when it's hard to be) +

I believe in forgiveness +

I love to laugh and like it when I laugh so much my cheeks hurt :) +

My mom's lasagna and spaghetti rocks +

I love football..especially the Steelers +

I love to play volleyball +

My family means everything to me +

I love my friends +

I love Hoss's and the Olive Garden +

I hate smoke +

3, 9, and 12 are my favorite numbers +

I love lattes especially French Vanilla +

I love jet skiing - the sand between my toes - staying up late and sleeping in +

I love small romantic gestures but I don't expect them +

I love surprises and surprising people +

I live to make other people happy (an impossible task, I know) and I always try to see the bright side of things (although it is really hard to do sometimes) +

I do have mood swings (hey I'm a woman) and they are pretty bad sometimes but that just makes it interesting +

I get instantly pissed when i get too hot or someone pinches me +

I don't like to hear gross things when I'm eating +

I have four brothers and three sisters and I love them all with everything I have and would do anything in the world for them +

I hate liars and dishonesty +

I believe in God and being loyal to those you love +

I have very little patience and probably too many pet peeves +

I love to sing loud and crazy when no one else is around and sometimes when they are +

I love to watch movies +

I love that feeling of complete and true happiness +

I hate losing friends, especially ones that have been a part of my life for a long time and mean just as much to me as my family +

I hate when people don't take the time to listen to other people and automatically assume they are right +

I get embarrassed easily +

I hardly ever yell at someone but when I do, I feel horrible about it and apologize even if I was right +

I don't like when people are mad at me +

I love to go on vacation and my dream is to make it to Ireland some day +

I hate when my friends are sad and there isn't anything I can do to make them happy +

I hate when people drink and drive +

I think crying is ok +

I think that when someone offers you unconditional love in the form of a friendship it should never be refused because there aren't too many people out there that will give it to you and truly mean it +

I love the holidays and the food that goes with them +

Don't be afraid to ask for help +

Dream big +

Work Hard +

Play +

Live * Laugh * Love

This writing was found on Katy's computer after her death. It was dated October 31, 2006, one day before the first anniversary of her transplant.

The Gift of Life

Excerpt of an undated tribute by Katy to her sister Shelly

Knowing my sister would risk her life for me when she has two beautiful daughters and a wonderful husband is something that I thank God for every day. There is no greater gift than the gift of life and that is exactly what she gave me. We always have been close sisters but when you go through an experience such as this one, a bond forms that no one and nothing can break.

After the transplant I remember how much pain my sister was in and I would always pray that somehow all of her pain would transfer over to me. I cried when I thought of how much she must love me to do this for me with such risks and how unfair it was that she was miserable. Since my transplant we have spent more time together than we ever did before. I spent most of the summer with her and her family. Both of our lives transformed into ones of appreciation and understanding. I can now live my life as a healthy young adult because my sister is an extraordinary person. I try to do everything in my power to make sure that she knows how much I appreciate what she did for me. I know that not everyone would risk so much and it takes a special person to give part of themselves to save another person but my sister is one of those special people.

She is my angel and there isn't anything I wouldn't do for her.

Acknowledgements

PITTSBURGH – When I was a boy growing up in San Juan, Puerto Rico, I watched my grandfather type on his Smith-Corona typewriter. He'd tell me he was writing a novel and I'd stare in awe, wondering about the story he was telling as his fingers danced on the keyboard.

My grandfather's name was Carlos M. Suarez. We called him Papi Carlos. He inspired me to become a writer, even though he wasn't a writer himself. He just happened to love the written word. Papi Carlos died when I was twenty-three, but his love of writing – and journalism – remains with me today. I sat with him in the living room of his house in the mid 1980s, watching what was then a little-known cable network called CNN. He'd be amazed at today's technology.

As I wrote this book, I thought about Papi Carlos, wondering what he'd think of Katy, Starzl, organ transplantation and the developments of modern medicine. He would have loved every aspect of this story. His passion lives in me and I thank him from the bottom of my heart for all he taught me in my young years.

As the years went by, in Puerto Rico and later in Pittsburgh, many people came into my life – some expected and some not. They supported me, cheered me, guided me, watched me, and above all, allowed me to become who I am as a writer and as a person. I'm sure some of them don't realize the impact they've had on my life.

My mother Isabelita – Papi Carlos's daughter – has always been my constant cheerleader and guardian. That's what mothers are supposed to do, but my mom faced a mountain of challenges as a single parent. She taught me to be fair, honest and fearless. When I became a reporter, I mailed her newspaper clippings and she always read them, even if she knew little about the subject matter. She taught me to be courageous and to respect the medical profession. I inherited from her a deep appreciation for people who are genuine and sincere. I wouldn't be where I am today without her by my side.

People constantly ask me why I don't live in Puerto Rico. I tell them my homeland is always with me and I am proud to be Puerto Rican. But not long after graduating from Duquesne University, I met a woman who would change my life. My wife, Jenny, is the reason why I stayed here. She fell in love with me and never questioned why I didn't make a lot of money. She read early drafts of the book and gave me the type of feedback only true friends can give – blunt and unapologetic. My wife's love is reassuring, inspiring and impossible to live without. She gave me a son and daughter – Daniel and Maria – who have been relentless in their support of this book. For weeks at a time, I'd come home from work, eat dinner, and sit at my laptop. Daniel would ask if I was working on "the book." If I chose not to sit at the laptop and watch TV instead, he'd ask "are you going to work on your book tonight?" Maria would follow, always asking when I'd be done. Probably never, I said many times. My kids inspire me to be a better person every day. They teach me, more than I ever teach them. By having this book in their hands, I hope they realize they need to work hard to accomplish their dreams. Very hard.

Many relatives, friends, colleagues and teachers have stood by me throughout the years: My brother, Enrique; my uncle Carlos; my aunts

Rosa Luisa and Zulma; my father, Fano, who would have preferred that I write a crime novel and always gives me sincere advice; my stepfather, Hector, who gives me guidance, motivation and makes me laugh until I cry; my late grandmothers, Mami Isa, who taught me that "God is always watching" and whose laughter I miss every day, and Abby, who never missed a chance to share her love of books; my English teacher at Colegio San Ignacio, Christine Noya, the first person to recognize my love of writing; Maggie Patterson of Duquesne University, who shared amusing tales of journalism; Eileen Spear, my first boss at Duquesne University's Campus Ministry Office; and Suzy Whelan, who is like a sister to me and, after more than twenty-five years of friendship, always finds a way to make me feel better about life's problems.

In my professional life, I have been fortunate to work with the best in the field – editors, reporters, and even public relations professionals. I was lucky to have Trish Hooper as one of my first editors. She was younger than me, but listened to me and, quite honestly, managed to figure me out in ways that no one ever did. Thank you, Trish, for those long chats we always had in your office. Bob Fryer, who hired me at the *Valley News Dispatch* and became my editor at the *Pittsburgh Tribune-Review*, made sure I was always accurate. He taught me that we're all bound to make mistakes and "if you're not having fun, you shouldn't be in this business." During his cancer treatments in 2010 and 2011, I sometimes drove him to work. I told him about the book and he confessed he was envious he never had a chance to write one. He died last year and would be incredibly annoyed if he knew that I miss him.

My newspaper work would not have succeeded without a lineup

of mentors: Rick Monti, Jim Cuddy, Julie Cryser, Dave Williams, Sandy Tolliver and the incomparable Jim Wilhelm. And of course, there's Frank Craig, the top editor at the *Tribune-Review*. He has nurtured me and believed in me, even though he knows every one of my flaws. His office door is always open. He listens and for that, I am forever grateful. The publisher of my newspaper, Dick Scaife, has given my colleagues and me the opportunity to create a competitive force in journalism at a time when the field is changing at an incredibly fast pace. His support of strong, serious journalism is part of a magnificent legacy.

In the fall of 2008, I began to do research about liver transplantation for a potential story about transplants in people who didn't need them. It was a complex subject matter, one that required an enormous amount of time and research. I talked to Fryer about it and we both agreed that I needed help to be able to accomplish what we needed to do. Pick any reporter you want, Fryer told me. The choice was a no-brainer. I chose Andrew Conte because I wanted to work with the best reporter I knew. Andy and I spent months working on the series, often cooped up in a windowless room for more than ten hours at a time. He was a workhorse, always one step ahead of me, always providing the time and insight that can only make a story better. To my surprise, I gained not only the benefit of his journalistic integrity but also a close friend. Only someone like Andy would grab me by the shirt while running Pittsburgh's half-marathon and literally pull me as I struggled to keep running. Only someone like him would read early drafts of this book and have the guts to tell me I could do much better. I've been lucky to have by my side someone who is ridiculously righteous and extremely loyal.

When I was near the finish line, Jennifer Bails edited the manuscript and inspected it line-by-line. Just like the times when we worked on projects together at the Trib, she made my words crisper and my grammar sharper. She is an excellent editor and one of my faithful supporters. My friends Robert Amen and Jeremy Boren helped with the tedious task of proofing and provided much needed creative advice. I am humbled by their talent. John Schisler not only gave me support, he also put up with my incessant complaints. Mel Wass shared her creative genius and time and produced a beautiful cover design.

A book like this one, with medicine and science as a backdrop, must be accurate and true to medical history. For their medical expertise, and for their commitment to the truth, I thank Drs. Ngoc Thai and Kusum Tom.

To say thanks to Dr. Starzl would seem insufficient. The best way to show my appreciation is to celebrate the lives of the people he saved with his tremendous talent. What an amazing life he's had.

It would have been impossible to tell Katy's story without the help of her family. I spent many hours on the phone with Kathy Miller, often going over the same things time and again. Often through tears, she displayed a level of patience I have never encountered. The same goes for Katy's dad, Roger, her brothers, sisters, and sister-in-law Martina. Shelly put up with my relentless questions, even though I always made her cry when she talked about Katy. I hope she and the rest of the family know that Katy's spirit will live with us for a long, long time.

Luis Fabregas

August 2012

About the Author

L uis Fabregas is an award-winning, medical journalist based in Pittsburgh. Over more than two decades working in the health care field, including thirteen years as a medical/investigative reporter for the *Pittsburgh Tribune-Review*, Fabregas has written about hospital infections, health care economics and organ transplantation.

His 2001 series, "Hannah's Story," about a five-year-old girl with terminal cancer, and his 2005 special report, "Born to Fight," about a couple who lost one of their premature twin babies, received first-place writing awards from the National Association of Hispanic Journalists. His 2008 series, "Transplanting Too Soon," co-authored with journalist Andrew Conte, received a first-place award from the Association of Health Care Journalists, the Carnegie Science Award, the 2009 top investigative prize from the National Association of Hispanic Journalists and several state journalism awards.

Fabregas earned a master's degree in communications and a bachelor's degree in journalism from Duquesne University in Pittsburgh. He lives in Natrona Heights, Pennsylvania, with his wife and two children.

CPSIA information can be obtained at www.ICGtesting.com
Printed in the USA
LVOW072131281012

304818LV00008B/244/P